DOCTORS, DILEMMAS, DECISIONS

Dedication

This book is dedicated to Dr Sunny Ebrahim, a supportive and loyal partner, and an outstanding general practitioner.

Doctors, Dilemmas, Decisions

Ben Essex, MBBS, MRCP, MSc, FRCGP

General practitioner
Honorary Research Fellow, UMDS Guy's and
St Thomas' Medical School, London

BMJ
Publishing
Group

© BMJ Publishing Group November 1994

First published in November 1994
by the BMJ Publishing Group, BMA House, Tavistock Square, London WC1H 9JR

British Library Cataloguing in Publication Data

A catalogue record for this book is available from the British Library

ISBN 0-7279-0859-6

Typeset, printed and bound in Great Britain by Latimer Trend & Company Ltd, Plymouth

Contents

Foreword

It has been said that general practice is both the easiest and the most difficult of medical specialties. It is easy to practise superficially and inadequately but extremely difficult to practise well in all its dimensions because these are so extensive.

The general practitioner is required to make decisions in every consultation and to do so in the average practice every eight minutes and on some 8000 occasions in the course of a year. The quality of care that a general practitioner provides therefore depends on the quality of decision making and the ability to encompass a full range of relevant issues in that compact and compressed process.

Ben Essex is a highly respected general practitioner trainer and course organiser and has acted as an adviser to the World Health Organisation, for which he produced important teaching aids for the training of health workers in the prevention of disease in developing countries. In addition to his wide interests and work in the field of mental health and in medical education, he has made a particular study of decision making in general practice and has published widely on this theme.

This book reflects his style, of introducing the reader to an understanding of decision making using logical processes. These allow the practitioner to encompass a full range of the issues to be considered in the management of patients in general practice. He shows his extensive experience and knowledge of general practice in his practical examples of clinical situations that help to develop a logical structure in decision making. The newcomer to general practice may be surprised to discover how wide ranging these issues are, whether they relate to interpersonal relationships in the consultation, a knowledge of the Children Act or to the provision of transport services for the disabled. The student of general practice, therefore, will find this book a most useful guide to understanding and practising the discipline.

I am happy to commend this book for use by general practitioner trainees, trainers, course organisers, as well as principals in general practice, and it should be a standard reference in postgraduate and practice libraries.

A G Donald
President, RCGP
1994

Preface

There is nothing new about making decisions in general practice but attempts to understand how such decisions are made are new. This is uncharted territory and one that is difficult to study. It is often assumed that because judgement, intuition, and experience are the basis of good decision making, these skills cannot be taught. During the past few years many new methods have been developed to study decisions made by doctors. This has resulted in the development of effective decision support systems in many fields of medicine. Such methods have not previously been applied to decision making in general practice.

The focus of this book is on how decisions are made. It is the study of process and not outcome. The total emphasis is on discovering the "best" route. Whether the chosen destination was reached or not is a secondary consideration. To make decisions that are ethical, cost effective, safe, and acceptable is all that can reasonably be asked of a general practitioner. To do so, many factors need to be considered. Each decision must be tailored to the specific problems, needs, and goals of the individual patient. Judgement is fallible, knowledge and skills are often deficient, and outcomes are never certain.

Over many years I have recorded and analysed thousands of cases from which "rules of thumb", forming the basis of intuition and experience, have been identified. The book is a selection of cases from patients who presented to me, my partners, and to nursing and other colleagues over the past 12 years. This book presents problems for students and trainees to consider, discuss, and formulate their own ideas about how they should be managed. It enables them to benefit from my own experience expressed in the rules presented in each case exploration. A partnership needs to be forged in which roles, responsibilities, and decisions are shared by doctors and their patients.

The research undertaken to study decisions in general practice is in its infancy. It is hoped that this book provides some insight into how intuition and experience are acquired, and how these might be utilised by students and trainees. These are exploratory beginnings. The readiness is all.

B ESSEX
1994

Acknowledgements

I am extremely grateful to my patients, without whom there would be no book. They have provided the experience and insight which form the basis for many of my ideas about decision making in general practice.

Many of the "dilemmas" were presented to us by our patients during the past ten years, and I am very grateful to my partners Drs Jackson, Ebrahim, Graver, Platman, Sikorski, and Thomas for their help in clarifying ideas about their management. Other cases were brought to my attention by colleagues who knew that I was interested in the decisions such problems represented and I value their contributions.

I appreciate the help that other specialists have given, especially Mrs Brenda Harris on cases and rules relating to the Children Act, Mrs Chris Smith on nursing issues, Mr Norman Ellis on employment dilemmas, and Dr Surinder Singh on problems relating to people with HIV/AIDS.

The book is based on a research project funded by the Primary Care Development Fund of the South East Thames Regional Health Authority. Dr Rodney Turner and Mrs Leslie Elliot have been a constant source of help and support at all times. I am grateful to Dr Stuart Handysides for his criticisms.

I would also like to thank Mary Banks and the editorial staff for their help in editing the book to ensure that it is as concise and clear as possible.

B ESSEX
1994

I Decision analysis

1 Introduction

Why study decision making?

A busy doctor makes hundreds of decisions every day, some of which will have a major impact on the lives of patients and their families. The ways doctors make decisions are not apparent to students and there is a feeling that it is intuitive. Learning from experience does not always lead to "good" decisions and may be distressing for patients and traumatic for learners. Bad experiences are not always recognised as such, and wrong lessons may be learned.

Doctors lack ways to reveal the thought processes behind medical decisions. Uncertainties abound and judgement is affected by many factors. Little work has been done to try to classify the many kinds of decisions that doctors make or the thought processes that lie behind them.

We learn from experience; this has to be interpreted, put into the right context, and incorporated into ethical and other value judgements—then it can provide a valuable guide to future decision making.

It is not surprising that undergraduates are not taught analyses of decision making in general practice given the lack of methods for teaching such skills. We can no longer rely on experience or hope that learning from mistakes will suffice. We need to find ways of teaching students and doctors how to make carefully thought out decisions about diagnosis and management.

Aim of the book

The aim of this book is to help students and doctors to make decisions that are ethical, safe, and acceptable to patients. It is hoped that it will help to answer the questions

What decisions need to be made?

Who should make them?

In what order should decisions be made?

What factors should be considered?

How should uncertainty be dealt with?

What is the optimal sequence for making management decisions about certain problems, for example, cot death, sectioning a patient, child abuse, etc?

How can doctors share decisions with patients?

What are the principles behind the delegation of decisions to others?

How should decisions be made when resources are scarce?

How can decision making skills be audited?

Medical students

Teachers of medical students

GP trainers

GP trainees

Practice managers

Non-medical people who are interested in professional judgement, for example, managers

Purchasers of services

---

that arise in reaching these decisions. Relevant questions are shown in the box.

Although written by a general practitioner, the broad principles and concepts outlined in this book are also applicable to doctors intending to enter other specialties. In addition, it could give managers and other interested groups some insight into the difficulties faced by doctors in making decisions about patient care.

Users of this book

This book is aimed at the groups of people shown in the second box although it has been written primarily for medical students and GP trainees, together with their teachers and trainers.

How to use the book

The way in which this book is used will depend on the educational goals of the reader. It may be read as a straight text, although some cases can be used to acquire management skills about specific problems. Teachers and learners may wish to explore certain topics, and the cases provide a focus for this. Although people learn in different ways, this book presents methods that can be used to enable them to learn about decision making in general practice.

Limitations

The reader may disagree with some of what is being presented; however, this could act as a stimulus to search for different, perhaps better, management options. This is not a "cook book" in which to find the "right" answer. It asks many questions, tries to explore the ways in which decisions are made, and is about the decision process itself rather than management outcomes. It is an attempt to analyse the "judgement" that lies behind decision making in general practice. Readers will bring their own unique experiences, interpretations, and disagreements to their reading of the cases, and this should help them to find alternative ways of thinking and deciding.

Basis of decision making

It is useful to think of a spectrum of methods used to make decisions: from intuition to scientific experiment. The GP uses qualitative and quantitative information before making decisions about the problems that present in daily practice. Sometimes intuitive judgements are used, and at other times decisions will depend on analytical ways of thinking, according to the nature of the task. A home visit to a temporary resident presents a relatively unstructured task where non-quantitative information will be assessed. Alternatively, when, for example, reviewing the liver function tests of a patient with hepatitis, quantitative information is being assessed.

Conclusion

In general practice decisions are affected by intitution, peer aided or consensus judgements, and data from epidemiology and controlled trials. An eclectic approach is needed. Intuitive judgements are often based on extensive experience and can be analysed to help students and trainees to develop decision making skills; this book tries to show how this can be done. The first step, however, is to identify a framework for classifying the types of decisions made in general practice.

2 Classification of decisions

Decisions in hospital and in general practice

There are differences in the way decisions are made by GPs and the way they are made by doctors working in hospital wards and clinics. These differences are shown in the table.

Decisions in practice and hospital

General practitioner	Hospital
Unselected problems	Selected problems
Decisions made in isolation	Decisions often made with other doctors
Fewer investigations to influence decision	More investigations affecting decisions
Decisions affected by knowledge about the family	Decisions often made without knowledge about the family
Less time available	More time to take history and do examination
Decisions about seriousness and urgency made outside hospital	Decisions about seriousness and urgency often already made
Minor and major illnesses	Predominantly major illnesses
Conditions seen at an early stage of the natural history of disease	Conditions seen at later stages of natural history of disease
Type and range of decisions very broad	Type and range of decisions more limited than in general practice
Decisions can be easily reviewed	Decisions more difficult to review after discharge of patient

In general practice a vast range of problems will be seen. These include the whole spectrum of physical, psychological, and mental illnesses, and their interactions with social and family problems. Considerable diagnostic skills are needed because of these multifactorial dimensions.

The GP works alone and often has to make difficult decisions without the opportunity of discussing it with a colleague. Most appointments are between 5 and 10 minutes and many decisions have to be made in this short period of time, including decisions about the need for diagnosis, investigations, treatment, follow up, prevention, and screening.

Decisions about the need for hospital referral or admission can be critical for many patients. Assessments of seriousness and urgency are often made early in the natural history of the illness before the patient is sent to hospital. Decisions would have to be made when the clinical picture is very different from that seen if emergency admission were needed.

As mentioned earlier, the type of decisions that GPs make are often different from those made by hospital colleagues: decisions about screening and disease prevention are usually made in general practice and not in hospital. GPs can ask patients to come back if symptoms have not resolved or get worse, whereas hospital doctors have more limited access to patients.

Decision framework

Prevention of problems

Identification of problems

Investigation of problems

Identification of management objectives

Selection and organisation

Management and follow up

Evaluation of outcomes (audit)

Prevention of recurrence

Daily decisions about patients seen in surgery and at home can be recorded, analysed, and used to produce a classification. The classification of decisions in the box is based on such a study;[1] it is empirical, pragmatic, and lacks any theoretical basis, but all the decisions relate to one or more of the tasks in the classification.

This classification is useful and helps to clarify the tasks undertaken in general practice.

Prevention of problems

Most patients who come to the surgery need some form of prevention or screening and these tasks can be a part of a consultation. In children, prevention of infectious diseases is a particularly important goal. In adults, prevention of cardiovascular disease and lung cancer should be part of every consultation. Patients can be screened for risk factors that could be reduced by changes in their lifestyles. Prevention of cervical cancer is an important goal and patients should be recalled for regular smear checks; women who are at risk of osteoporosis need to be identified. Prevention of HIV infection and malaria is of critical importance in certain groups of patients. Some acute problems can be prevented from recurring. Opportunistic prevention should be part of every patient encounter.

Identification of problems

The word "identify" seems to be more appropriate than "diagnose." Many patients have social, occupational, psychosexual, or domestic problems which may present as somatic symptoms. It is therefore more realistic to think about identification than about diagnosis, and about problems than about diseases. Doctors and patients may not have the same perception of the problem, and the same problem may be seen quite differently by different doctors.

Investigation of problems

Of all the methods available for investigation of patients the most potent of all investigative tools is history taking. Modern investigative techniques will enhance but never replace the skills of history taking. Decisions relating to investigations depend on the differential diagnosis, and the specificity and sensitivity of the tests themselves. If investigations are needed, then decisions must be made about their organisation and how the patient should be informed of the results.

Identification of management objectives

To answer the question "What am I trying to do?", management objectives need to be identified. Without clear management goals, outcomes cannot be assessed. Most patients expect doctors to have a clear idea of what the aims of prevention or treatment really are. If these are not clear, good compliance and shared responsibility are difficult to achieve. Stott and Davis[2] have identified the following four goals for every consultation: management of presenting problems; assessment of help seeking behaviour; management of continuing problems; and opportunistic health promotion.

Management of presenting problems

For the patient the acute problem may be of the greatest concern. There are, however, three other objectives to be considered.

Assessment of help seeking behaviour

The first thing to identify is whether the patient's response to the problem was appropriate. This can be ascertained by asking the four questions in the box.

The answers to these questions identify the need for education about appropriate help seeking behaviour.

Management of continuing problems

Coexisting chronic problems and treatment also need reassessment when a new problem arises. The interactions between acute and chronic problems and any medication involved may affect management decisions.

Opportunistic health promotion

Most preventive work in general practice is carried out in conjunction with management of acute and chronic illness. Every consultation presents an opportunity to achieve important goals related to screening and primary prevention.

Management selection and follow up

Once the management objectives have been identified, decisions need to be made about how these can be achieved. Examples of questions that should be asked are shown in the box.

---

1 Did the patient go to the accident and emergency department first?
2 Did the patient wait too long before seeking help?
3 Did the patient try self medication first, if appropriate?
4 Did the patient fail to recognise the seriousness or urgency of the problem?

What options exist?

Is there scientific evidence of effectiveness?

What are their risks and benefits?

What are the costs of alternative options?

What is most acceptable to the patient?

How should the management and follow up be organised?

What does the patient need to know about treatment and outcomes?

What follow up is needed and how should this be organised?

The answers to these questions will affect the decisions about management and follow up.

Evaluation of outcomes

There are several outcomes; possible ones are shown in the box. The responsibility for identifying these outcomes and taking appropriate action may be the GP's or the patient's, or it may be shared. It is important to be sure that these responsibilities are clearly defined.

Prevention of recurrence

This goal is often overlooked. Many patients have acute exacerbations of a chronic illness, such as asthma or colitis, and the management objectives should include prevention of recurrence wherever possible.

> Achievement of all the management goals
>
> Development of complications from treatment or illness
>
> Treatment failure
>
> Deterioration of condition
>
> Resolution of problem
>
> Failure to prevent recurrence

Conclusions

Each consultation involves decisions related to one or more of the tasks discussed above. This framework can be used as a guide to ensure that all the relevant decisions have been made and that no important decisions have been overlooked. It also helps us to analyse the management of individual cases. The use of a comprehensive framework always helps to clarify the way we think before we make any decisions. In chapter 3 we study how GPs make decisions in the surgery and during home visits.

1 Essex B. Decision analysis in general practice. In *Decision-making in general practice* (Sheldon M, Brooke J, Rector A, eds), London, Macmillan Press, 1985.
2 Stott N, Davis R. The exceptional potential in every primary health care consultation. *J R Coll Gen Pract* 1979;**29**:201–5.

3 Evaluation of rules

The rules presented in the cases throughout this book form a decision support system, but how effective is it when used by students and trainees? A research study was undertaken to evaluate the effectiveness of the rules developed by me over an eight year period.[1] A large number of vignettes based on real cases were selected for the study, covering a range of problems related to prevention, diagnosis, investigation, management, follow up, evaluation, and prevention of recurrence. They included ethical dilemmas, organisational and administrative problems, and problems relating to specific conditions such as HIV/AIDS, chronic illness, mental illness, and psychological and social problems. Each vignette had between one and seven rules judged by the author and assessors to be particularly relevant to that problem.

The participants comprised 93 fourth year clinical students and 191 GP trainees. Participants were each given four vignettes and asked to record their perceptions and management before and after exposure to a few rules. The participants' responses were judged by a panel of five assessors who were chosen to cover a range of medical opinion, and all of whom were experienced professionals. The results showed that the rules were effective in improving students' and trainees' perceptions and management decisions of "paper" patients.

A follow up study was carried out in which trainees were given new cases without any rules. The rules previously encountered were also relevant to these new cases, and the trainees were able to recall these rules even though there had been no attempt to memorise them in the initial evaluation some weeks earlier. This suggests that the rules are internalised and become part of the participants' conceptual framework.

The study showed that exposure to a few selected "rules of thumb" can improve the decision making competence of both undergraduates and trainees. The limitations of vignettes are recognised, and further studies need to be carried out to see if relevant rules are recalled when confronted with real patients.

This study shows that decision making skills can be acquired by the use of a rule based, decision support system. The next phase of this research is to undertake appropriate searches for the identification of the small number of rules relevant to any particular problem. Computer technology is ideal for undertaking this kind of search and also allows the rules to be amended and updated. Ultimately this type of decision support may become a standard feature for training students and trainees to develop decision making skills in general practice.

The reader may disagree with much that is presented, but it could lead to debate and discussion about the decision process itself, rather than the outcomes. The next step is to examine the many factors that affect decisions in general practice.

1 Essex B, Healy M. Evaluation of a rule base for decision making in general practice. *Br J Gen Pract* 1994;44:211–13.

4 Studying decisions in general practice

Decisions in the surgery

Most decisions about patients are made in the surgery where there is little time to analyse the decision process in depth. Case discussions focus on what was done rather than on how decisions were made. Video recordings show how well the patient and doctor communicate but the thought processes behind the management decisions are not seen or heard. Little research has been done to explore how decisions are made in general practice. Medical students often make decisions in an unstructured way, not recognising that decision making skills are essential and can be taught.

Decision support

How relevant to general practice are some of the more recently developed decision support systems? Statistical techniques, such as Bayesian methods, have been used to increase the accuracy of diagnostic decisions. Good statistical data may support an effective statistical program where the categories are small, overlapping, and are well defined. The inability to use qualitative knowledge limits the use of this approach in general practice, where problems are multidimensional and categories of diagnoses are not mutually exclusive.

In reviewing the literature of medical decision making in the last 20 years, I perceive a shift from dependence on observational data and a greater emphasis on "judgemental" knowledge, which reflects the experience and opinions of the expert. Qualitative experiential judgement can be described in so called "rules of thumb" which follow a line of reasoning as opposed to a sequence of steps in a calculation.

As decision making in general practice also depends on judgemental expertise, there is a need for rules or principles that operate even though the doctor may not be conscious of them. The challenge is to identify them and discover how they influence decisions. This is a difficult area of research as the methodology needed to explore complex intellectual tasks is in its infancy.

People called "knowledge engineers" are employed to identify the often subconscious rules derived from analysis of the ways in which experts make complex decisions in many fields, including law, medicine, biology, and chemistry. Cost and confidentiality make this approach difficult in general practice. Here, the GP is both the expert and the "knowledge engineer."

Decision research in general practice

In 1989 the Primary Care Development Fund of the South East Thames Region gave me a research grant to study decision making in general practice, the overall objectives of which are shown in the box. The methods used in this research study are outlined below.

Identify the types of decisions made in general practice

Identify the sequence in which decisions are made

Identify the factors that affect such decisions

Identify the "rules of thumb" that form the basis of judgement in general practice

Study the impact of these "rules of thumb" on the decisions of undergraduates and trainees

Case analysis

A brief record was made of selected cases and their management, and any obvious factors affecting the management decisions were also recorded. These notes were very brief and made immediately after the consultation had ended. A recent example is shown below.

Case 1

Woman aged 55 fell, fractured hip. Now recovered from surgical treatment. Given a certificate to return to work. Osteoporosis to be excluded. For bone density test and review.

Differential diagnosis

Risk factors for osteoporosis

Need for diagnostic tests

Prevention of recurrence of fracture

Need for follow up

Osteoporosis is a preventable disease and observations that enable women at risk to be identified include a history of:

- early menopause before age 45
- oophrectomy before age 45
- family history of osteoporosis
- previous fractures
- use of oral steroids   [764]

- Prevent problem
- Identify problem
- Investigate problem
- Determine management objectives
- Select and organise management and follow up
- Evaluate outcome
- Prevent recurrence

Later that evening, the case would be analysed while still fresh in the mind. The factors affecting decisions in this case included those in the box.

Could this fracture have been prevented if she had been given hormone replacement therapy? Were there risk factors that indicated a risk of osteoporosis? The "rule of thumb" that arose from this case is shown in the margin (764).

Over a ten year period thousands of cases have been analysed in this way. Although the research continued for over 10 years, the funding for evaluation has been provided during the last four years.

Classification of decisions

All decisions were recorded, analysed, and found to fit into one or more of the following tasks in the box. Each of these tasks involves making many different decisions. For example, when evaluating outcomes, the GP must decide on the points in the box on page 16.

Further analysis was carried out to classify the types of decisions made within each of these subgroups. This initial study resulted in the development of a framework for classification of decisions and identification of their sequences.

Whether such evaluation is necessary

Who should undertake this task

If follow up is needed and how it should be organised

What to tell patient about:
- follow up
- possible complications of illness or treatment

How to identify different outcomes

What to do if no better or worse, or if new problem develops

What to do if patient defaults from follow up

What observations to select to evaluate outcome

If outcome is successful, whether recurrence can be prevented and, if so, how

Whether an unsuccessful outcome is the result of a diagnostic error or the treatment being:
- inappropriate
- inadequate
- intolerable
- interacting with other drugs/ diseases
- incomprehensible to patient
- wrong because of administrative or organisational error or failure of communication
- not taken by patient
- aimed at inappropriate objectives
- based on a premature evaluation
- affected by a complication or development of a new problem
- ineffective in preventing recurrence

How an unsuccessful outcome should be managed

Identification of factors

Decisions in general practice are affected by many factors such as age, occupation, mental state, etc. The management of each problem was studied to identify the factors that affected management decisions in each case. These data were recorded immediately after each patient contact, and are given in chapter 5.

Definition of rules

The way in which the factors affected decisions are described in the "rules of thumb", an example of which was shown in case 1, where the rule related to risk factors for osteoporosis and the need for hormone replacement therapy. Over 800 brief "rules" have been identified by this research, most of which are not disease specific. For example, a diabetic patient whose blood sugar was very high on routine follow up was asked if she was keeping to her diet. She replied that she was doing so, "between meals."

This led to the following rule.

> In a diabetic whose blood sugar is high check compliance before evaluating effectiveness of treatment

This rule was specific to diabetes, but it also applied to the evaluation of other chronic diseases. Therefore reference to diabetes was removed.

> Assess compliance before changing medication, or evaluating outcome or effectiveness

The rule was no longer disease specific and could now be applied to any condition. Over 90% of the rules are not disease specific, but some do relate to specific problems such as child abuse, HIV infection, mental illness, etc.

The name "rule" sounds objectionable to most doctors but a "rule" based system consists of brief guideline statements. Such "rules" are not commands that have to be obeyed.

> **In this book, a "rule" is only meant to be a suggestion or guideline**

Most of the rules presented in this book, will be familiar to experienced doctors. The reader is free to reject or modify them whenever it seems appropriate to do so. However, those based on current national guidelines or new legislation should not be amended. References will be provided when they are based on new legislation such as the Children Act, Department of Health guidelines, or newly published evidence.

Priorities

> Reason for referral
> Social and family circumstances
> Severity of disability
> Urgency
> GPs' knowledge of other doctors
> Acceptability
> Waiting lists
> Economic factors
> Hospital resources
> Financial resources
> Time of year
> Referral guidelines

One of the most difficult tasks in medicine is the establishment of priorities. This is because they reflect value judgements and people do not share the same values. The priority of legal and ethical factors is easy to establish, but it is more difficult to be sure of the priority of other factors. For example, management decisions about referral are affected by some or all of the factors in the box. In what order of priority should these be placed? If there is no budget left to treat any more patients until the next financial year, the nature of the problem, its disability, severity, and urgency will all influence the decision about whether to consider other options, for example, extra contractual referral or private treatment. What is considered an "acceptable" wait? Somehow all these factors will be given different weightings dependent on the information available at the time. The difficulty involved will be analysed in the review of cases throughout the book.

From practice to theory

Most of the cases presented in this book are based on real problems that have presented to GPs over the last 10 years. Many of the theoretical concepts come from studying decisions made in daily practice,[1] with the rules being derived by the study of individual cases, the views of experts, scientific evidence, current guidelines, and new legislation. The important point is that analysis of real problems led to the development of the concepts and methods of decision support presented in this book. The critical question is whether undergraduates and trainees make "better" decisions when they have access to the rules presented in this book? A brief summary of the research undertaken to answer this question is presented in chapter 5.

1 Essex B. Decision analysis in general practice. In *Decision-making in general practice* (Sheldon M, Brooke J, Rector A, eds), London, Macmillan Press, 1985.

5 Factors and pathways

Factors affecting decisions

Decision making in general practice is affected by a large number of important factors, which are difficult to identify and classify. Below is a list of these factors; it is not comprehensive; the classification is pragmatic and lacks any theoretical basis.

Health problem

Differential diagnosis
Aetiology
Infectivity
Information accuracy

Natural history of illness
Objective findings
Probability of occurrence
Coexisting problems, past or present

Seriousness
Severity
Urgency
Duration

Patient

Acceptability
Age
Seen by appointment or as emergency
Risk factors
Behaviour
Risk of conception
Breast feeding
Immunological status
Defaulted from follow up
Self discharge
Violence or agression
Compliance
Cultural factors

Disability
Expectations
Perceptions
Past experience
Holiday imminent
Information, need for
Memory
Mental state
Nationality
Occupation
Pregnancy
Prejudices/values
Rights
Sensitivities/allergies

Social or family circumstances
Treatment, previous responses
Recently in the tropics
Recent bereavement
Financial difficulties
Child on protection register, past or present
Unemployment
Redundancy
Private health insurance
Ability to pay
Homeless
Advance directives

Family

Assessment of problems
History
Information needs

Problem impact on
Requests
Responses

Resources
Support
Social deprivation

Other people

Effects of problems on others in community
External pressures, requests
Person accompanying patient
Person who sent patient

Referral from one clinic to another
Responses or opinions of other
- people
- doctors

Trainee or student present
Neighbour support
Politicians
Patient participation group

Doctor

Assumptions
Communication difficulties
Experience past
Expertise/skill
Ignorance
Uncertainty

Knowledge
Mental state
Prejudices/values
Reaction to problem
Relationship with:
- other health personnel
- partners

- patient
- relatives

Workload
Time
Fear of litigation
Fund holding status
Conflict of interest

Investigations

Indications
Reliability
Results

Availability
Cost
Access
Contraindications

Interpretation/report
Knowledge of investigator, eg, radiologist
Guidelines

Resources

Budget available
Allocation
Priorities
Rationing criteria

Amount needed
Availability
Policy
- practice
- community

- hospital
- Department of Health
- regional or national

Cost effectiveness

Time factors

Day of week
Waiting list

Duration of surgery appointments
Duration of treatment

Time of day
Duration of illness or problem
Bank holiday

Medicolegal

Legal factors, eg, recent legislation
Guidelines
- specialist
- district
- regional
- national

- Department of Health
- UKCC laws

Ethical
- confidentiality
- rights
- autonomy
- informed consent

Power of attorney
Possibility of court case
Impending FHSA complaint
Political policies
Method of payment

Management

Administrative factors
Organisational factors
Indications for treatment
- initiating
- stopping
- continuing

Drugs
- current administration
- interactions

Cost effectiveness
Evidence from randomised controlled trials
Side effects
Probability of risk
Errors
Geographical factors

Objectives
Alternative options
Request for private treatment
Policies
Protocols
Practice formulary
Indications for allowances/ benefits
Carer's needs
Conflict of interests
Shared care responsibilities
Use of deputising services
Roles and responsibilities
Information available
Home visit
Ineffective traditional rituals

Availability
- beds
- surgery appointments

Purchaser contracts
Indications for extra contractural referral
Knowledge of hospital consultants
District nurses
- availability
- quality

Mistakes
Night calls
Opinions of
- consultant
- other colleagues
- district nurses

Many factors affect management decisions. Are some of these factors more important than others? Should some always be considered, whereas others only need consideration under certain circumstances? Do some conflict with others? The answers to these questions help our understanding of decision making in general practice.

Priorities

There may be a conflict of interest among several factors, all of which may be relevant to a specific problem. Relatives' requests may conflict with patients' needs and rights. There may be a conflict of interest between the rights of the parents and those of a child. The 1989 Children Act clarifies such issues. Confidentiality, informed consent, and other basic rights take priority over other factors most of the time. There are, however, exceptional circumstances when they should be overridden. Ethical factors apply in all cases but others, such as waiting lists, indications for treatment, etc, will only be relevant in certain cases. Some factors should therefore be considered before others. For example, it would be unwise to select the place of referral for surgery before assessment of whether or not the waiting list is acceptable. The sequence in which certain factors

21

are considered is very important, and acceptability should not be considered until the patient has all the relevant information about alternative options, waiting times, and quality of services. Careful professional judgement is needed to ensure that all the relevant factors are taken into consideration in an appropriate order, with recognition of their interrelationships and relative importance. The list of factors is not totally comprehensive. Readers will think of new ones to be added.

Identification of "rules"

The "rules" outlined in this book describe how factors affect our decisions.

> **A rule is a guideline which the reader is free to accept, modify, or reject**

When a rule is based on current legislation or national guidelines, references will be given. The reader is encouraged to identify rules included in this book. Others may of course lead to disagreement and debate. Remember the rules here are just suggestions, open to modification or to rejection.

Decision pathways

The management of certain problems can be analysed to discover the "optimal" operation sequence for tasks. Analysis of decision pathways can help to make management safer and more effective.

Death certification

There is an optimal pathway for decisions that need to be made when called to issue a death certificate. After confirmation of death, the history has to be established. The first thing to decide is whether the death can be certified by the GP, based on the observations in the flow chart.

Who can certify?

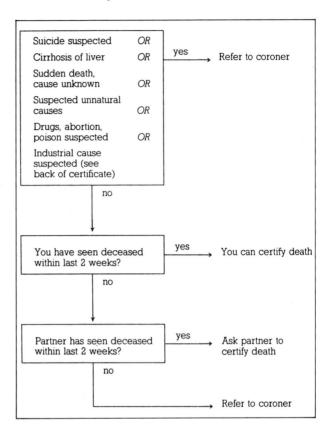

Coroner referral:

- inform family why this is necessary
- explain procedure
- telephone coroner.

AIDS and death:

Death certificates are not confidential documents and families are sensitive about this cause of death. You need to decide whether to state cause or to indicate on the certificate that further information would be made available on request to the Office of Population Censuses and Surveys, and to the Centre for Communicable Diseases.

Death expected:

Within days If about to go on holiday ensure that partner in practice sees patient before death to prevent an unnecessary referral to coroner.

Within hours Give relatives your home phone number. Decide whether they should telephone you, if death occurs at night, or notify you in the morning.

Death occurs

When confirming death in the night, relatives should be asked to come to the surgery in the morning to collect the certificate. If death occurs during daytime the procedure is as follows.

Notes, forms

Takes notes, death certificate, cremation forms, and practice leaflet for relatives explaining procedure.

Examination

Examine body.

Organ, body donation

Did deceased indicate organ or body donation? If so eyes must be removed within six hours if corneas are to be donated. Contact eye hospital. If body has been donated contact HM Inspector of Anatomy. If death has to be reported to coroner, his or her permission must be obtained before organs or body is donated.

Death certification

- Sign the death certificate.

- Put in envelope.

- Detach notice and give to informant.

- Find out which relative intends to register death.

- Show the information needed by registrar listed under duties of informant.

- This information, death certificate, and deceased's medical card to be taken to registrar.

- Give address of registrar.

Children

Have they had a chance to see the deceased before removal of body? If appropriate discuss with family.

Pacemaker

If present decide if you wish to remove it and claim the fee. If not, inform the undertaker who will do it. Explain to family that this has to be done if body is to be cremated.

AIDS, hepatitis

Undertakers should be told to take special anti-infection precautions. Consider confidential reporting to communicable disease surveillance centre.

Cremation

Explain that another doctor must examine the deceased. If family agrees to body remaining in house until second doctor arrives, complete your part and give form to relatives to give to second doctor. If they want body removed, find out where it will be. Contact second doctor who must be fully registered for five years, and not a practice partner. Give details.

Sedation

Assess need and provide sedation if necessary.

Follow up

Give a follow up appointment for relative to come to the surgery after the funeral. This is the best time to assess needs as initial family support may have been withdrawn.

Inform others

Others who need to be informed may include practice partners, district nurses, hospital, hospice, health visitor, social services, and surgery staff. Ensure that any further outpatient clinic appointments are cancelled. Inform Family Health Service Authority (FHSA) if in recall group for cervical cytology.

Bereavement visit

Decide whether this is necessary or not and, if so, which practice partner should do it.

Refer to social worker

Decide if help is needed in getting death grant and coping with pensions etc.

Collect supplies

Doctor should collect drugs. Nurses usually collect their supplies and equipment.

Amend records	Remove from age–sex registers
	Enter on death register if these are audited.
	Enter bereavement on problem list of spouse and children.
Follow up	Follow up consultation to assess need for bereavement counselling and other support.
Return records	Enter date and cause of death in patient's record. Return to FHSA.

This decision pathway helps to ensure that important tasks and decisions are not overlooked. The sequence may not be "optimal" and you will have to decide for yourself whether it should be modified.

Sectioning patients

Criteria

A patient is suffering from a mental disorder severe enough to warrant detention in hospital for assessment.

The patient ought to be detained in the interests of his or her safety, and/or for the protection of other people.

Informal admission is not acceptable to patient.

Types of section

Section 2

This is for a 28 day admission. Treatment may be given without the patient's consent.

Section 4

This is for a 72 hour admission. Treatment can only be given with the patient's consent.

Section 3

This is for a six month admission for treatment.

Factors affecting decisions

The decision on what section to choose will depend upon a number of factors, including:

- past history of illness, previous relapses;

- previous response to treatment, severity of illness;

- urgency, risk of violence, family circumstances, time of day

- availability of other people, opinion of others;

- acceptability to family.

Forms and personnel

To admit under section 2, signatories are a section 12 approved psychiatrist or doctor, a GP, and either approved social worker or nearest relative. If section 12 approved doctor is not available, is delay safe and acceptable? If not then section 4 is the only option. Signatories are GP (or psychiatrist if he or she becomes available) and approved social worker or nearest relative. Note, for section 4, that patient must be seen by both signatories within 24 hours. Avoid asking relatives to sign unless there is no alternative.

Resources

Bed, access to phone, forms for sectioning patient, paper and envelopes, drugs, time, transport, people including relative, social worker, psychiatrist, community psychiatric nurse if known to patient, and police if necessary.

PROCEDURE

The following procedure relates to section 2 but it includes actions to take should section 4 be selected. A complex series of decisions has to be made and one possible sequence is described below.

Identify catchment

Determine if patient lives in hospital catchment area. If in London telephone the Emergency Bed Service. Give patient's address and ask for psychiatric catchment area. If daytime, phone psychiatric hospital and ask duty senior house officer or psychiatric secretary. If not in catchment area you will be told which hospital to contact. If in their area ask which duty psychiatrist would carry out a domiciliary visit to assess need for sectioning.

Telephone duty psychiatrist

- *Can carry out domiciliary visit:*

—arrange time to meet at house. If you cannot be there, arrange access, inform relatives, friends, or neighbours
—contact approved social worker (see below).

● *Not available today:* Will psychiatrist be available tomorrow? Consider following factors: urgency, severity of disturbance, past history of admission and outcomes, effect of delay on family, risk of violence to self or others. If it must be today, admit under section 4. Only use section 4 if there is unacceptable delay in undertaking a section 2.

● *Delay acceptable:* Sign your part of form 3.

Leave it with relative or friend of patient or in the practice and inform social worker where it can be collected.

Ensure family can be contacted by telephone and told time of psychiatric visit.

Arrange for social worker to visit and collect forms.

Medication Avoid intramuscular medication before psychiatrist and social worker have had a chance to assess patient.

Telephone social worker Telephone social service department or town hall if out of hours. Speak to social worker who deals with sectioning patients. Discuss case and ask for home assessment by social worker. Arrange for joint visit if possible. If not, ensure social worker has access to patient. Arrange where and when to discuss case afterwards. Inform if risk of violence.

Disagreements If there is a disagreement between you and the social worker about need for sectioning, do not get angry. Identify reasons for disagreement and practical alternatives. Consider social worker's views carefully. If you do not change your mind:

● Ask social worker to provide a written report on reasons for not sectioning patient.

● Ask social worker to give the relatives a telephone number to contact again if new problems develop.

● Record your opinion on the appropriate form which is valid for 5 days.

28

- Leave form with patient's relatives and, if situation alters or social worker changes his or her mind, it can then be signed.

- Write a factual account of what has happened and any adverse outcomes, and keep a copy in the patient's record.

Reassessment

If there is a delay or disagreement about the need for sectioning, it should be reassessed the following day. Relatives are asked to report any new problems that may necessitate immediate reassessment. Inform practice partner on duty, that night or the next day, of the situation.

Organising admission

- Telephone hospital to confirm bed available.

- Write referral letter.

- Check all relevant forms have been completed.

- Enclose them with referral letter.

- Social worker will accompany patient.

- Give letter to whoever accompanies patient.

- Consider police support:
  —if necessary: telephone to confirm arrangements;
  —ask police to wait at a discreet distance until ambulance arrives.

- If necessary arrange for removal of young children from house, before ambulance arrives to avoid psychological trauma.

- Explain to children what is happening and why.

- See if they can stay with relatives or friends.

- Order ambulance.

- Ensure you or social worker or both stay with patient until ambulance arrives.

- Ask relatives to let you know what the outcome of admission is, and when patient is being discharged.

- Enter illness episode on patient's problem list

- Ensure patient is put on the practice mental illness disease register

- Claim fee for sectioning patient.

Decisions about what to do and in what order to do them can be critical when patients are being sectioned. "Getting it right" can reduce the trauma and the time taken to admit the patient to hospital. It reduces duplication of effort, and clarifies the roles and responsibilities of all involved. Can you identify a better decision pathway?

Summary

In this chapter we have tried to identify some of the many factors that affect decisions in general practice, and begun to explore the concept of "critical pathways." Making "good" decisions means considering the most relevant factors and identifying all the decisions that need to be made. The importance of identification of the "optimal" sequence in which decisions should be made is clear, and this concept can be applied to the management of many other problems in general practice. The next task is to identify who should share in the decisions that need to be made about patients and their management.

6 Training

Patients have to pay a high price for any failure on the part of medical schools to teach decision making skills to students. This book tries to show the importance of this skill in general practice. Competency based training must be developed to enable these skills to be acquired. Teachers have to be convinced of the need for such training and make use of new methods to help students and trainees make "good" decisions in general practice.

Curriculum

Few medical schools include courses on decision making in their curriculum. It is assumed that students and doctors will develop these skills by learning "on the job." Some do, but many do not. An early introduction to decision making is appropriate as a subject of universal application to all disciplines within medicine, and is in fact relevant in many fields, including ethics, sociology, epidemiology, law, behavioural science, and the evaluation of scientific evidence. Teachers and students must decide whether or not decision making skills should be an educational goal. A self instructional computer module may overcome the difficulties of fitting yet more topics into an overcrowded curriculum.

Methods of learning

Computer

I am currently developing the software necessary for development of a self learning programme to develop decision making skills in general practice. When completed it will contain menus for 25 chronic diseases, the rule based expert system, 350 cases, and a learning package. This will be available to interested teachers and course organisers.

Games

MEDILEMMA is a game designed by me to explore the factors that affect decisions in general practice. Course organisers and trainees have found it a valuable training tool and great fun to play.

UDUNNIT is another game designed to explore decisions related to iatrogenic problems in general practice.

Both games can be obtained from me on request.

Role play

Many of the problems presented in this book can be used in role play, and people can add their own dilemmas to those already described. This is ideal for multidisciplinary teaching as many of the cases involve several members of the primary care team.

Case analysis

Problems encountered in daily practice can be used to examine the types of decisions made, and the factors taken into consideration. This case analysis approach can be used to test the validity of the rules themselves, or to develop new ones.

Rule base

The rules presented in this book have been selected from a larger set. A software program exists to search this database for the two or three rules relevant to any specific problem. It also allows the rules to be modified or updated as needed. Students and trainees can use the rule base when they need decision support, whether in relation to prevention, problem identification or investigation, selection of management goals or options, follow up, or prevention of recurrence.

Factor analysis

Decisions can be reviewed to discover whether the most relevant factors were considered. The priority given to different factors in the final management decision can also be identified, with the focus on the decision making process and not management itself.

Specific problems

Some topics, for example, mistakes, staff, or children's problems, can be used to analyse decisions that depend on knowledge of legal aspects of our work such as employment law or the Children Act.

Perceptions

Trainees can compare their perceptions of problems with either those of others or those of their trainers. They can also analyse the decisions made by the consulting doctor. Video-recordings can be used to identify decisions that were:

- observed to be made;

- thought about but considered inappropriate;

- overlooked but should have been made.

This analysis can be done using one of the decision frameworks presented in this book; decisions that the observer perceived as being made are recorded and compared with those that the doctor thought were being made. Patients may have a quite different perception of these decisions, and these can also be studied.

Modifications

Many of the "rules of thumb" outlined in this book will probably sound like commonsense, but students may not recognise when they are relevant to other problems. Teachers and students can develop new rules and modify others. Some of the rules will change over time, as new laws or guidelines for ethical practice are provided. A workbook could be constructed in which new cases could be added, and others updated or revised.

Menus

Options for management selection for 24 chronic diseases have been shown to provide valuable decision support for trainees and experienced doctors. At present, these are available from me in paper format.

A total of 211 cases are analysed in this book and they are numbered consecutively. The rules are randomly selected from a large set and their numbering is not sequential. I hope that teachers will want to train undergraduates and trainees to acquire decision making skills. They will use whatever methods seem most appropriate to their needs. Such techniques are non-threatening and provide a clear basis for changing decisions without a sense of failure.

7 Sharing decisions

Doctors are in an unequal partnership with their patients. It is both possible and desirable for them to share decisions, but in practice, there are many obstacles that make this difficult to achieve.

Sharing power

- Sharing decisions about which management goals to select
- Improved compliance
- Clear division of roles and responsibilities
- Shared accountability for outcomes

Doctors can exert great power over their patients as a result of their professional experience, knowledge, and skills. It is controlled by a mixture of paternalism, high technology, and secrecy over the ways in which diagnoses are made, treatments selected, and ignorance hidden. Many doctors now recognise the advantages of sharing the decision taking with their patients. This implies shared accountability, which has not been fully recognised by patients. The real limits of "shared care" relate to our willingness to share power with patients, relatives, and carers. Its advantages include those in the box.

Power sharing leads to a recognition of limits and an admission of uncertainty.

Sharing information

The key to power sharing is the ability to share information and ignorance with the patient. In medical schools the skills valued by role models exclude that of imparting information to patients in a way that is clear, concise, comprehensive, comprehensible, accurate, relevant, rational, and non-judgemental. The GP has to help the patient to find the right questions to ask and this can be a difficult task.

Presenting information

Responses are determined by the ways in which information is presented. Your glass is half full, can I get you another drink? Your glass is half empty, can I get you another drink? These presentations invite different responses. All information contains bias. However, ways of presenting information that help patients to make more informed decisions need to be studied.

Case 2

A man aged 51 has cystinuria and has developed another renal stone. This has been treated with lithotripsy which has broken up the stone almost entirely. The consultant haematologist writes to say: "I discussed the long term treatment of cystinuria and said there were two alternatives. First, he could continue on his previous regimen of high fluid intake and with luck he would make very few stones. He has sometimes had gaps of up to 15 years between stones. If he did develop a stone, however, it could be treated with repeat lithotripsy or open operation. The other option is that he has penicillamine to prevent stone formation. This would involve taking up to 1000 mg eight hourly for the rest of his life. He will think it over and come and see me after his next lithotripsy."

Sharing decisions of this sort with the patient involves giving all the information needed to make an informed decision. The letter does not mention the risks or effectiveness of the pencillamine treatment. The GP may not have this information but the patient could be helped to identify the most relevant questions. These include asking about the probability of more stones forming, the acceptability of lithotripsy treatment, and the effectiveness and risks of long term penicillamine treatment. These questions should be written down. The haematological and renal side effects of penicillamine could be looked up in the *British National Formulary* and discussed in the surgery. The haematologist or urologist might be able to answer questions about the effectiveness of this treatment. The patient could defer a decision for a while, as there are no more stones present.

Sharing uncertainty

Doctors are often uncertain about what to do for their patients. This is understandable considering the lack of data about the effectiveness of the many therapies used.

35

There are few well conducted and conclusive, randomised, controlled trials on cost effectiveness of alternative treatments. If decisions are to be shared doctors have to share their uncertainties with patients. Many doctors believe that expressing doubts about management decisions would undermine patients' confidence but it may increase the respect people have for their doctors. It seems acceptable to express uncertainty when trying to obtain informed consent but not at other times.

Sharing management decisions

There is clear evidence that management outcomes improve when patients are taught about the significance of their symptoms and what to do when their condition deteriorates. For example, prescribing peak flowmeters without a system of self management and regular review will not improve the care of asthmatic patients.[1]

Sharing decisions with patients means sharing responsibilities for bad outcomes. Sharing decisions about objectives, management, and follow up are key elements in shared care. It clarifies the roles and responsibilities of both for maintenance of health, treatment of illness, and prevention of recurrence.[2]

Shared care records

These have become well established for diabetic patients, but are not so well recognised for patients with serious mental illness. In a pilot project that I undertook, 84 schizophrenic patients held their own shared care records over an 18 month period. Doctors had to be taught how to write information that was accurate and acceptable to the patients. They were encouraged to record the patients' own words such as "still afraid that people are listening to thoughts at night" rather than use terms such as "deluded."

Patients were enthusiastic about holding their own records. They valued being consulted about what was recorded, and found the record of their treatment and progress useful. Patients felt it made it easier for them to challenge their doctor. Many psychiatrists, however, felt threatened by this approach, even though it has been shown to improve communications among health staff and facilitate the identification of potentially dangerous drug interactions.

Shared care records were acceptable to patients with severe mental illness; they increased their autonomy, and improved communication and effectiveness of shared care. Obstacles to further development of this approach relate to the attitudes, perceptions, and anxieties of the doctors, nurses, and managers. These can be overcome if the advantages of sharing decisions and power with the patients can be recognised.[34]

Role models

Students need models on whom to base their future behaviour. Research has shown that, in general practice, the trainer is the most powerful role model for the trainee. It is from such teachers that trainees learn the skills needed to empower patients and to act as their advocates.

Advance directives

This is a method for ensuring that patients' wishes are respected when they are unable to provide informed consent. Consider the following case.

Case 3

Man aged 41 with severe multiple sclerosis is looked after at home by wife and district nurses. He is extremely weak, now unable to feed himself or to hold his head up for any length of time. He has had two episodes of pneumonia, the last of which involved being put on a ventilator for two days. The nurse asks what you intend to do if he develops another pneumonia. "Would you treat him doctor?" What is your response?

> It is the competent patient's right to be involved in any decision about investigation, treatment, or place of care
>
> [224]

Should the GP discuss this with his wife before he develops another chest infection? If she asks that antibiotics be withheld would you agree to this request? If she says "it's up to you doctor" what would you do? What is the ethical issue in this case? (224)

37

> Good management may include creating opportunities for patient and family to discuss fears, and wishes about death and dying [618]

> What do you feel about your illness?
>
> What aspects of life still give you pleasure?
>
> What are your thoughts about the future?
>
> What frightens you most?

> Doctors and relatives ought to respect requests about terminal illness management made when the patient was competent and these may be clarified by advance directives [439]

The problem for the doctor is how to involve the patient in such a decision (618).

Useful questions include those in the box; they allow anxieties and fears to be expressed. The patient may wish to talk about dying. Patients often want to ask the doctor "how will I die," and yet feel embarrassed about doing so (439).

An opportunity must be created to enable this patient to discuss all these things. He may then express his wishes about the degree of treatment for any pneumonia. These should be recorded in the records for other doctors to see.

Interactive video programmes

Such programmes are available to supplement the opinions and advice of specialists. Patients can watch an interactive video programme[56] that explains the causes of the disease, its symptoms, outcomes, and the risks of each treatment option. They have direct access to the results of clinical trials and patient surveys, together with first hand accounts from previous patients. These are now available for patients with prostate problems, hypertension, low back pain, and early stage breast cancer. The Kings Fund Centre is evaluating these videos.

By presenting all the available information, the videos make decisions that are truly shared by doctors and patients a real possibility. The combination of videos and personal computers enables patients to select information relevant to their personal circumstances. The information is presented in a format that is easy to understand. How many specialists would be comfortable using such techniques to empower patients and facilitate informed choice?

Delegation to patient

Doctors delegate many decisions and responsibilities to patients.

Tasks delegated to patients

Identification of relapse, complications, side effects, or deterioration

Taking appropriate action when these problems arise

Prevention of recurrence, correct administration of treatment

Self monitoring of illness, assessment of urgency and severity

Deciding when to call or consult the doctor

Factors affecting successful delegation of tasks and responsibilities

Clarification of responsibilities and tasks to be delegated

Agreement about what is to be delegated

Provision of the necessary knowledge and skills needed

Review of competence; provision of adequate resources

Having realistic expectations of what is feasible

Provision of clear, comprehensible, concise, written instructions

Provision of backup support when uncertain

Audit of the outcome of such delegation

Clarification of the legal and ethical issues

Factors affecting the decision to delegate tasks

Acceptability, competence, feasibility

Degree of backup support available

Family, social, and cultural factors

Resources available, type of problem

Ethical and legal implications

Availability of medical or nursing support

Wishes of patient or family

Delegation can lead to power sharing if all these factors are considered and acted upon. Only then will doctors be in partnership with their patients.

Conclusions

Sharing decisions with our patients should be part of daily practice. Unfortunately it is a skill that has to be learned, and not something that can be taught by experience. Many factors need to be considered, and new legislation affects daily practice and patient expectations. Different methods have been developed for helping doctors and patients to be more effective in sharing decisions. We need information about the cost effectiveness and acceptability of new techniques so that we can select those most appropriate for any given situation. This is a new field but opens up new possibilities for real partnerships between doctors and patients.

1 Charlton I, Charlton G, Broomfield J, Mullee M. Evaluation of peak flow and symptoms on self management plans for control of asthma in general practice. *BMJ* 1990;**301**:1355–9.
2 Grampian Asthma Study of Integrated Care (GRASSIC). Integrated care for asthma: a clinical, social and economic evaluation. *BMJ* 1994; **308**:559–64.
3 Essex B, Doig R, Renshaw J. Pilot study of records of shared care for people with mental illness. *BMJ* 1990;**300**:1442–6.
4 Shared care of patients with mental health problems. Report of a Joint Royal College Working Group. Royal College of Psychiatrists and Royal College of General Practitioners. Published by Royal College of General Practitioners, Occasional Paper 60, 1993.
5 MacLachlan R. An out and out success. *Health Service Journal* 1992; **102**:26–7.
6 Ellwood PM. Outcomes management: a technology of patient experience. *N Engl J Med* 1988;**318**:763–71.

II Specific decisions

8 Diagnosis

In general practice, many conditions present at an early stage in their natural history and the initial diagnosis is usually made without the help of other doctors. In hospital several doctors see the patient and will contribute to the diagnostic debate. They will also have access to a wider range of investigations.

There has been a surge of interest in decision aids and the ways in which doctors make decisions. Throughout clinical medicine, there is increasing evidence of poor decision making which can be improved by the sensible application of formal decision techniques. De Dombal[1] points out that diagnostic accuracy among inexperienced doctors is falling. For acute abdominal pain it is 35–40% in the UK, among the lowest in Europe.[2] The lead time from presentation to a doctor with symptoms, which are subsequently shown to be the result of caecal cancer, to firm diagnosis is around 48 weeks. One in eight patients with a cardiac problem presenting to an accident and emergency department has been seen somewhere else and sent away.[3] There is now good evidence that when the results of formal decision aids and detailed scrutiny of clinical decisions have been sensibly introduced into routine clinical practice, there follows improvement in performance, particularly among inexperienced staff. In relation to acute abdominal pain, Adams showed that, when findings of detailed studies were made available to inexperienced staff, performance improved in a number of hospitals.[4] The application of similar decision support to the diagnosis and management of acute chest pain greatly improved diagnostic accuracy. Similar analysis reduced the lead time from presentation of gastrointestinal cancer to firm diagnosis from a median period of 24–52 weeks to 30 days.[5] The argument that decision analysis is unrelated to performance ignores a significant body of evidence. In general practice, a good differential diagnosis must include less common but more serious conditions.

Case 4

A man aged 48 worked as a teacher in East Africa until six months ago. He feels well but coughed up a small amount of blood a week ago. There is no pain, dyspnoea, sputum, fever, weight loss, or cough. He stopped smoking a year ago. There are no abnormal findings on examination. He is taking children on a school holiday in two days' time and will be away for 10 days. What is your management?

This man feels well and is about to go away for 10 days. Are further investigations needed? The possible alternatives include those in the box.

Referral for bronchoscopy

Referral to the chest clinic

Recall for another radiograph in three months

Reassure him but ask him to return if there is a recurrence

Investigate in the practice, with full blood count, sputum examination, etc

It was decided to send the patient for a chest radiograph, which was normal. If a carcinoma is, however, present, this is the time when surgery can be curative. He may not have a recurrence of haemoptysis for some months, by which time the carcinoma could be inoperable. What is the likelihood of his having a small carcinoma of the bronchus? (118)

More information about the probability of serious underlying disease or complications may help to decide if further investigations are indicated [118]

Each doctor will have a different risk "threshold" for undertaking further investigations. Some would consider that further tests are justified if the risk of a carcinoma was as low as 5%; others might accept a probability of 10%. Is such information available? (491)

In a patient with haemoptysis and a normal radiograph, the probability of malignancy is 9% and further investigations are indicated
JAMA 1988;**259**:1333–7 [491]

Without these facts there is considerable uncertainty. Is it reasonable to decide not to request a bronchoscopy without discussing it with the chest consultant? (399)

An event may have a low probability of occurrence, but a high probability of serious consequences to patient and others, and this affects decision to investigate [399]

Who has the right to make this critical decision? Should the doctor allow the patient to decide on the need for bronchoscopy or is this a matter of "professional" judgement? The patient could be given relevant information about the probability of an underlying carcinoma. There is a risk in undertaking any invasive investigation, but there is also a risk that, by not doing so, a potentially curable cancer will be missed (116).

Follow up is no substitute for investigation to diagnose treatable cancer if malignancy is suspected [116]

Does the patient have the right to participate in the decision whether or not to undergo bronchoscopy? One way in which he could be told is: although the radiograph is normal there is still a 5–10% risk of a small tumour. The

| Choice of specialist |
| Place of referral |
| Urgency |
| Method of referral |

only way to be certain of excluding this is to pass a tube so that it is possible to look directly into the airways. Is the patient willing to accept a 90% certainty of no tumour, or would he prefer to be 100% certain? This man was a smoker until a year ago and this risk factor also needs to be considered. If it is decided to refer him for bronchoscopy the decisions that now need to be made relate to those in the box.

These decisions are affected by the resources needed and the waiting list for surgery. Should the receptionist make the appointment or should a letter be sent requesting an urgent appointment? This decision will depend on how urgent the problem seems to be. A two week delay could be prevented if the receptionist makes the appointment and this would ensure that it is within an acceptable period of time. If a letter is sent, should the patient be told what to do if his appointment exceeds a specified period of time? Decisions should be made on the assumption that he might have an operable carcinoma of the bronchus.

Case 5

A woman aged 82 is a temporary resident staying with her granddaughter. She normally lives alone and copes well. Two weeks ago her granddaughter found her confused and disheveled. She brought her back home hoping that she would improve but she has deteriorated. She is now incontinent, smelly, dirty, and does not recognise familiar people. The granddaughter says that she cannot possibly cope and asks you to organise for her to be taken into care. What is your management?

| The aetiology of abnormal behaviour must be identified before appropriate management decisions are made [111] |

| Diagnosis of abnormal or irrational behaviour should be based on direct interview and observation of the patient, and not just on evidence from a third party [110] |

Is this a housing problem? Is it a social problem because the relative cannot cope? The relative and the doctor may well have different perceptions of this problem. It affects social and family life, but is primarily a diagnostic problem (111, 110).

> Reversible causes of delusional and confusional states must be excluded before assuming that it is the result of senile dementia
> [112]

> Always exclude a physical cause for abnormal behaviour [135]

> Management decisions about long term placement in care should be made after treatment of acute illness if present [136]

Why is this patient behaving in this way? (112 and 135)

On examination she was found to have pneumonia. The granddaughter agreed to supervise the treatment and the district nurse was asked to visit (rule 136).

Decisions about long term care were deferred until the pneumonia was treated. She responded well to the treatment and her mental state returned to normal within 10 days.

Case 6

A man aged 51 telephones to say he has had an attack of palpitations which lasted for 30 minutes when his pulse was 116/min. It made him sweat but there was no chest pain or breathlessness. It has now gone. Three weeks ago he was discharged from hospital after a cardiac bypass operation which was complicated by a cardiac arrest; he spent two days on a ventilator. He says that his pulse is now 80/min and regular. He feels very well and is taking a daily dose of aspirin. "Should I worry, doctor?" What is your response?

> If symptoms have subsided and signs are normal, management decisions must be based on differential diagnosis, risk of recurrence, probability of serious illness and outcomes, and availability of emergency medical treatment [199]

> The differential diagnosis of a problem arising after recent discharge from hospital includes a complication of the treatment or illness, and should be discussed with relevant hospital staff [522]

What factors affect management decisions when symptoms and signs are normal? (199)

The GP's decision may be of critical importance to this patient. He has undergone major surgery, followed by serious complications that required intensive surgical and medical care. It could all be for nothing if the wrong decision is now made. The type of arrhythmia cannot be identified as it has now subsided. When a problem arises soon after discharge from hospital the safest approach is to share the management decision with the hospital specialist (522).

The cardiac registrar in this case felt that the patient ought to be admitted and monitored for 24 hours. It is important to distinguish those decisions that should be shared with others from those that GPs are competent to make alone. Patients are reassured when their doctors seek appropriate advice from hospital colleagues.

Case 7

A woman aged 38 complains of weight gain and anxiety. Her husband runs a pub and she feels that she should help, but since his accident she has a fear of crowds. Two years previously he had been assaulted by a customer with a glass and his median nerve was severed. This was unsuccessfully repaired leaving the hand severely disabled. His wife has to help him do up buttons etc, and the marriage has been severely affected by this accident. She seems depressed and unhappy. What is your management?

Some problems can only be effectively identified and managed by interviewing the patient's partner or children [470]

The severity of a problem and its disability should be assessed in functional, psychological, occupational, social, and sexual terms [176]

In making management decisions, disability assessment may be more important than diagnostic labels [177]

The GP and patient must decide whether to accept a consultant's opinion on diagnosis or management, or seek a second opinion [202]

This case seems to be about the way this couple's relationship has been affected by the accident (rule 470). How can the severity and disability of such a problem be assessed? (176)

It takes time to assess this kind of problem and a joint interview with both partners could be undertaken outside surgery time. The management objective would be to assess the problem, and to identify management options rather than to provide any treatment. This woman did not feel that this would be acceptable to her husband. The assessment of her husband's physical disabilities is relevant to the management of their problems (177).

Her husband's notes were examined later. The orthopaedic surgeon's last letter stated that there was no possibility of further repair to the severed median nerve (202).

Does the GP accept the consultant's opinion or not? Much depends on knowledge of the particular surgeon. Was he a hand specialist? Were reasons given for this opinion? Sometimes a second opinion can be obtained by telephoning a specialist to discuss the case. This ensures that the consultant's opinion is obtained and may prevent an unnecessary referral.

A consultant who specialised in hand surgery was telephoned; he felt that it should be possible to repair the nerve. The husband was asked to come in to discuss what else could be done for his hand. A second opinion was suggested and accepted. The couple were also referred to the practice counsellor. The operation resulted in full restoration of function to the hand nine months later.

This was accompanied by a great improvement in their relationship.

This case highlights the importance of considering the social and psychological effects of disability on two people, and not just on the person who consults the doctor. It also shows the need to consider the evidence upon which the consultant's opinion is based.

Case 8

A woman aged 54 has intermittent diarrhoea with mucus but no blood, which has been present for the last three weeks. She is not incapacitated but is anxious about this. There are no abnormal findings. What is your management?

If the differential diagnosis includes treatable malignancy, investigations should be done if the patient is fit enough to withstand tests and treatment [117]

The differential diagnosis is important and includes infections, inflammatory bowel disease, and malignancy. It is tempting to wait and see if symptoms resolve, as they often do, even if the underlying cause was a malignancy. However, the symptoms may recur a few months later by which time the growth could have spread (117).

Infectious or parasitic diseases should be considered in the differential diagnosis of problems such as diarrhoea and fever, and enquiries should be made about recent visits to the tropics [196]

The differential diagnosis includes infection with amoebiasis or *Salmonella* sp., so stool samples should be sent (196).

Doctor's management decisions are affected by patient's occupation [207]

This patient has not been abroad, and the duration of her symptoms made a neoplasm or colitis more likely than a bacterial or parasitic condition. Another relevant factor is the patient's occupation (207). This patient is a cook and was advised to stop work until an infective cause had been excluded. Where the differential diagnosis includes infection, inflammation, or malignancy, infective causes should always be excluded. If there is no evidence of infection, further investigations are needed to exclude malignancy.

Case 9

A man aged 57 presents with haematuria and is found to have a carcinoma of the bladder which has been treated with surgery and deep X-ray therapy. The prognosis is thought to be good. He feels well and requests a certificate to return to work. He asks you why this growth should have developed. What is your response?

When making a differential diagnosis occupational factors may be relevant   [213]

A diagnosis of "cancer" describes pathology but not the aetiology, for which other explanations should be sought (213). This man had worked for 15 years in the cable industry. How relevant is this to the type of cancer he has developed? (461)

An expert opinion is essential to make an accurate diagnosis of an occupational disease   [461]

A specialist in occupational medicine should be consulted because there are legal and financial implications to such an occupationally induced disease.

Case 10

A woman aged 76 has glaucoma treated with eye drops. Three months ago she presented to the trainee with an anxiety state caused by her fear of going blind. On examination there was no deterioration in vision. The trainee reassured her and prescribed lorazepam. Six weeks later she attended hospital and was told that the pressure had risen and that she needed tablets as well as drops. She is distressed by this deterioration and asks why this happened. What is your response?

This patient presents with a severe anxiety state which relates to her eye condition. There is no evidence to support her fears about going blind, but it is very difficult to reassure her, and she has been put on an anxiolytic medication. The ophthalmologist observes a rise in pressure and deterioration in her glaucoma. A differential diagnosis of the reasons for this deterioration must be made (43).

Assess patient's compliance before evaluating outcome or effectiveness   [43]

Patient's compliance is the first thing to check in elderly patients who may forget their medication. She was, how-

The diagnosis of the cause of deterioration in a chronic illness includes iatrogenic conditions [229]

In problem identification and differential diagnosis, always consider drug side effects, interaction, or withdrawal [279]

When evaluating outcomes, deterioration may be the result of recent drug treatment for a new illness, rather than failure of current therapy for the chronic disease [552]

The GP should inform hospital staff of any changes in medication in a written note given to the patient to take to clinic [551]

Before selecting a drug or continuing to prescribe it, consider its possible effects on pre-existing or current diseases [228]

In patients on long term medication who develop new symptoms or signs, it is important to diagnose whether it is caused by a drug, a known illness, or a new problem [283]

ever, taking the treatment at the right times and in the correct way (229).

Could an iatrogenic condition be relevant in this case? (279, 552)

GPs and hospital doctors often change treatments without informing each other. This results in increased morbidity and sometimes mortality (551). Before lorazepam is prescribed, its contraindications should be considered. Even though the doctor may know about the drug/disease contraindications, the problem often arises because they were not considered before selection of treatment (228).

In this case an error occurred because the possibility of interactions was overlooked. Decisions about contraindications must precede decisions about therapy, as the sequence of decisions taken can be critical to effective management.

Case 11

A woman aged 53 has intermittent abdominal pain for three months. Her husband is out of work and they have one son who is in an open prison. She has a past history of long standing depression, with occasional psychotic features. There have been several suicide attempts and she has been on amitriptyline and chlorpromazine for years. She does not drink alcohol. On examination she is jaundiced and tests show grossly abnormal liver function tests. She refuses hospital admission because her son would abscond from prison if he knew she was in hospital. What is your management?

Admission to hospital was advised to diagnose the cause of her jaundice. Unfortunately this was not acceptable. What is the differential diagnosis?

This problem has arisen in a patient who is on long term medication (283). What interactions should be considered in a patient who has a chronic illness and develops a new disease? There are two diseases and two different treatments. Possible interactions complications or side effects are the following:

- disease A/disease B

- disease A/treatment A

- disease A/treatment B

- disease B/treatment A

- disease B/treatment B

- treatment A/treatment B

> When treating one disease in the presence of another, consider disease interactions as well as drug interactions [186]

Could the drugs used for the patient's mental illness (disease A) have caused the jaundice (disease B)? Chlorpromazine can cause jaundice. Does the hospital know that she was taking this medication? (186)

> Long term medication may need to be changed when an acute illness develops in a patient with a chronic disease [185]

Should the patient continue to take medication or are these drugs contraindicated in liver disease? (185)

This case illustrates the need for good communication between hospital and general practice. It is worth finding out if her son would be allowed to visit her in hospital, as this could make a difference to her decision not to be admitted.

Case 12

A man aged 51 is seen at home with renal colic and admitted to hospital. Discharge note says IVU showed a stone in left ureteric orifice. He has a urological follow up appointment in two weeks. He feels well. What is your management at this time?

The diagnostic "label" should identify the aetiology of the problem and not just describe physiological or pathological states [282]

Some labels may reflect a physiological state, for example, cardiac failure, anaemia, renal stones, pulmonary oedema, atrial fibrillation, pleurisy, etc but do not describe the underlying pathology or diagnosis [479]

Is this a diagnostic problem or not? The "diagnosis" of a renal stone is inadequate (282, 479).

A proper differential diagnosis includes conditions such as parathyroid disease, and further investigations such as urate and calcium levels are indicated. These are often overlooked by the hospital staff, and it is the responsibility of the GP to ensure that they are done.

Should the patient be given any treatment or not? He is now asymptomatic but he could develop renal colic at any time. Do you want to visit him at night if necessary or would you prescribe some diclofenac for him to take should the pain recur?

Case 13

Neighbours are very worried about a lady aged 83 and they ask you to visit. She lives alone, has no relatives, is very deaf, and just sits in the window all day, picking at a piece of cloth. She looks miserable and complains of feeling "lousy" and having headaches. She looks depressed and there is a past history of her taking an overdose eight years previously. She has not seen a doctor for six years. On examination there are no abnormal findings. A full blood count, erythrocyte sedimentation rate (ESR), thyroid, and urine tests are all normal. She has meals on wheels and a home help, but has refused an offer to attend a day centre. She has no television or radio. You arrange for the psychogeriatric team to visit. They prescribe anti-depressants which she does not take. You revisit and she is sitting in the same place. What is your management now?

Disability caused by deafness includes depression and social isolation [377]

What is happening to this woman? Is this a diagnostic or a social problem? Could they be connected? (377, 376, 378)

Deafness is often a coexisting problem that needs assessment and management, for example, in patients with learning difficulties and in elderly people [376]

Management of deafness includes diagnosis of its cause and assessment of indications for hearing aids, home modifications, and other communication aids [378]

This patient's mental state improved greatly after her ears were syringed and the very hard wax was removed. She was then fitted with a hearing aid which helped to restore communication.

Case 14

A man aged 68 presents with enlarged glands in neck and has normal blood tests and chest radiograph. He is referred for a biopsy which showed a lymphoma. He refuses conventional treatment and tries homoeopathy for six months. He becomes very ill and finally accepts admission to the oncology unit. His wife now telephones to say that after four days of treatment he has discharged himself as he did not like the nurses. He accused them of using oxygen and poisoning his food. "Just thought you should know what has happened doctor." What is your response?

Hospital staff should immediately inform GP about self discharge of a patient with a potentially serious illness [510]

First hand information from hospital is essential for effective follow up of self discharged patients [46]

When an acute mental illness occurs in patients being treated in hospital for a serious physical illness, and the patient decides to self discharge, a drug induced illness is probable and acceptability must be reassessed after home treatment [509]

The most significant observation is that this patient was rational on admission to hospital and is now paranoid. This should be seen as a diagnostic problem and the cause of his delusional state needs to be identified (510).

The hospital staff have not informed the practice of his self discharge (46).

Information about his treatment is very relevant (509). He had been treated with large doses of steroids and was given these drugs to take home. His delusional state was drug induced. When the steroids were stopped, however, his mental state returned to normal. Acceptability must be considered in the context of the patient's mental state, and this should always be reassessed after treatment of a serious mental illness. Other treatments for the lymphoma were accepted once the paranoia had resolved.

Case 15

A woman aged 78 calls for a home visit because of severe difficulty in swallowing. Ten days before she had finished a course of radiotherapy for superior vena caval obstruction secondary to carcinoma of the bronchus. Dysphagia has been present for a week and is getting worse. At present she vomits a lot and even finds it difficult to swallow fluids. "Please don't send me back to hospital doctor." What is your management?

Is this about acceptability or is it a diagnostic problem? (62) Effective management in this case depends on accurate identification of the cause of dysphagia (522).

Could treatment have caused the dysphagia? The most likely diagnosis was oesophagitis as a complication of the radiotherapy. She was treated with cimetidine and her symptoms rapidly resolved (599).

This problem could have been predicted. It is a common complication of radiotherapy, and prophylactic treatment could have prevented much discomfort. Alternatively she should have been given clear instructions on what to do if this symptom developed (95).

Information given to patients should be specific and needs to be written down (472). Leaflets ought to be developed together with GPs. This is a subject that could be discussed by the GP representative to the relevant clinical directorate.

Patients are often told to contact the hospital if there are problems. If help is needed, however, it is most often sought from the GP. A leaflet could identify the areas of shared care and responsibility.

Case 16

A woman aged 26 is a new patient who gives a history of ulcerative colitis for six years. She says she is under hospital care but has to travel to Leeds to sort out divorce and custody of the children. There are no old records. Her diarrhoea is bad at present and she requests prednisolone (Predsol) enemas and codeine phosphate. You ask for details of the hospital where she was recently admitted to request a recent summary, and she gives the name and

---

A differential diagnosis of a new problem must be made before assuming that it is caused by a pre-existing illness [62]

The differential diagnosis of a problem arising after recent discharge from hospital includes a complication of the treatment or illness, and should be discussed with relevant hospital staff [522]

The complications of some treatments can be predicted and prevented [599]

Information given to patients, relatives, or other observers should include how to identify complications of recent treatment and what to do about them [95]

Ill patients who are being managed at home, and their relatives, need information about:

- what to do
- how to identify complications
- what to do about them
- when to call the doctor
- what to do if no better in specified time or if worse
- when the doctor will revisit [472]

ward. You write but they do not reply. She is seen by different partners on four more occasions. Once, when she said she had recently been admitted, the hospital ward was telephoned but they had never heard of her. A hospital consultant's secretary was asked to forward a summary but this never arrived. Recently, she came to see the trainee having had an emergency colostomy which he confirmed was working normally. This was done in a private hospital in Leeds but there is no discharge note. She said she did not want this operation and was very sorry it had to be done. Her parents paid for surgery but she could not remember the name of the surgeon or details of which hospital she was in. She is well oriented and not at all confused. She asks for another prescription for her prednisolone enemas and codeine phosphate. What observations do you make about this case so far, and what is your management at this time?

This is the case of the "therapeutic decoy". It is bizarre and difficult to understand, yet all the clues were there from the beginning. She has attended several times for a repeat of her medication (594). Many unsuccessful attempts have been made to get information from hospitals and previous doctors (722). There is no evidence to support a diagnosis of colitis, and yet she is being given prednisolone (Predsol) enemas and codeine phosphate (723).

How might codeine addiction be related to her recent operation? (283)

It may be necessary to obtain urgent information about new or temporary patients from previous GPs, other hospitals, or the Department of Social Services [594]

Requests for medication need to be supported by objective diagnostic evidence of the disease for which the drugs are being prescribed [722]

The diagnosis of drug addiction should be considered in a patient who makes repeat requests for medication but in whom there are no clinical observations, old records, or statements from previous doctors to support a chronic illness [723]

In patients on long term medication who develop new symptoms or signs, it is important to diagnose whether it is the result of the drug, a known illness, or a new problem [283]

> The differential diagnosis of illness in a new patient who has made repeated requests for medication should include the side effects of addictive drugs, including codeine   [724]

A differential diagnosis should be made in this case. The patient has objective evidence of recent surgery. Is the assumption that it was done for colitis justified? (724)

If this patient were a codeine addict she might have had the colostomy as a result of drug induced faecal obstruction. When confronted with this possibility she became very angry and left the surgery. She was never seen again. It took a long time to realise that codeine addiction was the diagnosis. The "therapeutic decoy" made it less obvious.

Case 17

A Ugandan bible student aged 26 complains of clumsiness in using the right arm. She also has some pins and needles in the right leg. These symptoms have been getting worse over the last six weeks. On examination she has normal sensation and power, and there are no other abnormal findings on neurological examination. She has always been in good health and there is no past history of serious illness. What is your management?

> In an African patient with unusual neurological symptoms or signs, the differential diagnosis must include encephalopathy secondary to AIDS   [693]

Multiple sclerosis is very rare in Africans. She was referred to the neurologist but two weeks later she returned because she was at times unsteady on walking. There were no new findings. She was seen in the neurology clinic that week. The consultant telephoned to say that he thought that it was hysteria but he would admit her for further investigations (693).

The diagnosis of encephalopathy secondary to AIDS had not been considered by the GP when she was first referred. Later on the consultant said that it was his first thought, but he had dismissed this possibility as her last sexual contact had been 10 years previously. She had never had a blood transfusion or any injections in Africa. She died of AIDS encephalopathy within eight weeks of admission. The long incubation period of HIV infection should not be overlooked.

Diagnostic criteria

How many psychiatrists in the UK use the same definition of schizophrenia? Do most obstetricians use the WHO definition of gestational diabetes? There is a need to agree on diagnostic criteria for certain conditions. A doctor's diagnosis will have profound effects on the social, psychological, and occupational life of a patient. The failure to standardise diagnostic criteria leads to many disagreements among doctors and to inappropriate treatment. Examples of diagnostic criteria include the WHO definitions, DSM-III-R and ICD-10 diagnostic classifications for mental illness, and the Read classification. Failure to use standardised diagnostic criteria could have profound implications for decisions made by doctors, patients, and their families.

Conclusion

Diagnosis is multidimensional and includes the psychological, social, and medical components of a problem. Diagnostic skills can be refined by the use of the many powerful new methods available. Teachers should not feel threatened by computer techniques or rule based systems. They should consider these as ways to refine our own diagnostic skills. Hopefully some of the approaches that they present can be intellectualised so that we acquire what seems most relevant to our needs. The message can be acquired without the media.

Once a decision has been reached about what the differential diagnosis might be, the next decision is whether or not further investigations are needed.

1 de Dombal FT. In *Analysing how we reach clinical decisions*, chap. 1 (Llewelyn H, Hopkins A, eds), London, Royal College of Physicians, 1993.
2 Pera C, Garcia-Valdecases JC, Grande L, de Dombal FT. European Community acute abdominal pain project meeting report, 1991 Barcelona. *Theoretical Surgery* 1991;6:188–91.
3 Emerson PA, Russell NJ, Wyatt J, *et al*. An audit of doctor's management of patients with chest pain in the accident and emergency department. *Q J Med* 1989;70:213–20.
4 Adams ID, Chan M, Clifford PC, *et al*. Computer-aided diagnosis of abdominal pain. A multi-centre study. *BMJ* 1986;293:800–4.
5 de Dombal FT. Computer aided decision support in clinical medicine. *Int J Biomed Comput* 1989;24:9–16.

9 Investigations

Every day decisions have to be made about the need for investigations, and how to organise and interpret them. Such decisions are usually based on the differential diagnosis. How would this investigation alter management? The answer to this question helps to decide whether the investigation is needed.

Case 18

A woman aged 38 has dysuria, frequency, and haematuria for three days. There are no previous episodes or abnormal findings on examination. What is your management?

This is a very common problem and decisions must be made about the necessity of treatment with an antibiotic. Options are shown in the box.

Decisions are affected by the past history, previous midstream urine results, and the day of the week. In this case it was a Monday morning, and the patient had no past history of urinary tract infection (31).

- Send midstream urine specimen and treat symptomatically until results obtained
- Send midstream urine specimen and then treat with antibiotics
- Treat with antibiotics without doing a midstream urine specimen
- Examine the urine
  —if clear give symptomatic treatment
  —if cloudy give antibiotics with or without sending a midstream urine specimen

An investigation is only indicated if it alters management   [31]

The management of a woman with haematuria and dysuria is different if investigations have excluded drug side effects, for example, warfarin or a urinary tract infection   [32]

Why send a midstream urine specimen if antibiotics are going to be prescribed anyway? If you did a midstream urine specimen and then gave antibiotics, how would the test result change your management? (32)

If the midstream urine specimen was sterile, further investigations would be needed after establishing that the blood was really in the urine and not coming from the vagina.

Case 19

A man aged 32 has epigastric pain which wakes him at night and is relieved by food. It has been present for a month. He has never been ill before. On examination he was tender in the upper abdomen, and he is not clinically anaemic. He does not smoke or drink alcohol, and his stools are not black. What is your management?

In problem identification and differential diagnosis, always consider drug side effect, interaction, or withdrawal   [279]

Should this patient be investigated, given symptomatic treatment, or treated with anti-ulcer medication? What is the differential diagnosis? (279)

Urgent investigations are needed in a patient who has recent onset of dyspepsia which can be drug induced   [179]

He may have a chronic illness and be on long term medication with a drug that could cause peptic ulceration. In such a case the diagnosis has implications for long term therapy (179).

If he had recently developed temporal arteritis and was on steroids, the decision to confirm the presence of a peptic ulcer may have important implications for the type of steroid preparation prescribed and for long term treatment with anti-ulcer drugs.

Management decisions are more critical at weekends and bank holidays as available resources are limited at these times   [2]

Should anti-ulcer treatment be reserved for patients in whom the diagnosis has been established? If so, many patients will have to be investigated. In a patient of this age, with typical ulcer symptoms, it seems reasonable to prescribe anti-ulcer drugs without endoscopy and to reserve investigations unless there is a relapse after treatment. Would you agree with this? How would an investigation alter management? It may be Christmas Eve or the patient may be about to go on holiday (2).

The decision to investigate is affected by time, day, occupation, coexisting diseases, current medication, patient's holiday plans, and disability, as well as differential diagnosis [588]

Identification and management of stress is as important as drug treatment in the management of peptic ulcer [94]

Information given to patients, relatives, or other observers should include how to identify complications of recent treatment and what to do about them [95]

The decision about fitness for work pending investigations depends on:

- occupation
- risk to others and to patient if symptoms recur
- current disability
- natural history
- differential diagnosis
- risk of spread of infection
- risk and severity of complications
- legal requirements
- occupational guidelines
- past history [567]

Current treatment might influence the decision to investigate. If he was on warfarin this might affect this decision. Age and past history will also affect present management. A haemoglobin of 10 g would increase the probability of a peptic ulcer causing occult blood loss. This would affect the management decision (588).

Another important factor is recent mental stress which may be a precipitating factor in patients with dyspepsia (94).

Follow up should include instructions on what to do if problems or complications develop (95).

This patient should be told how to recognise signs of a melaena or haematemesis, and what action to take if a bleed occurs. The decision to investigate should not be made until all these relevant factors have been considered. The decision to investigate would also be influenced by the patient's occupation, as it has to be decided whether he is fit for work (567).

This patient was an airline pilot. Should he be advised to stop work or to continue? How can the risk to others be assessed? The advice of an occupational health specialist may be useful. There may be strict regulations about flying under such circumstances, and further information is needed. Occupation is a very relevant factor but is often overlooked. GPs and local gastroenterologists could identify acceptable guidelines on indications for endoscopy, which would make effective use of a scarce and expensive resource.

Case 20

A man aged 62 coughed up a small amount of blood on one occasion. There were no abnormal findings and the chest radiograph was normal. He was referred for bronchoscopy. Two weeks later he returned to say that bronchoscopy had revealed nothing, but a special series of radiographs showed a tumour. He was prepared for surgery, but the night before the operation the consultant looked at the radiographs and disagreed with the senior registrar. He felt that the films did not show a tumour and there was no need for an operation. The next day he was discharged. No letter has yet been received. The patient is bemused, relieved, and slightly confused by it all. What is your management?

Is this a diagnostic problem or does it relate to the investigations that were done? Management options include those shown in the box.

- Reassurance of the patient that there is no serious disease
- Advice to return if haemoptysis recurs
- Referral elsewhere
- Repeat of radiology in eight weeks
- Discussion of the case with hospital staff
- None of the above

Disagreements about interpretation of an investigation should be resolved by discussions with the experts concerned   [122]

When diagnostic problems arise in spite of hospital investigations, direct discussion may avoid repetition of costly and uncomfortable investigations   [63]

Decisions will depend on the perception of this problem. This patient was admitted to investigate the cause of his haemoptysis and he was investigated appropriately. The problem relates to the interpretation of an investigation. There is a disagreement between the surgeon and the radiologist about whether the special radiographs showed a tumour or not (122).

It is always preferable to discuss the disagreement with the experts rather than to refer the patient to another hospital (63).

In this disagreement it is the radiologist who is the expert and not the surgeon. The GP telephoned the radiologist to discuss the radiographs. The radiologist was sure that they showed a tumour and said that he would discuss the radiographs at his weekly meeting with the surgeon. A week later the surgeon wrote to say that he had reconsidered the case and would be seeing the patient in the clinic to explain that there was a tumour and surgery was needed. The patient had a successful operation for a carcinoma and died of a coronary thrombosis seven years later.

Case 21

A woman aged 37 comes to surgery at 6.30 p.m. complaining of pain in her left calf muscle for three days. It came on over a period of one hour and has remained constant ever since. There is no past history of serious illness. She has been working and gets pain on walking, but she has no chest pain, cough, or dyspnoea. On examination there is mild tenderness in the calf muscle but no oedema or swelling. She is not on the contraceptive pill or any other medication. She does not smoke. What is your management?

The differential diagnosis should include more serious conditions which may need to be excluded before more common conditions [18]

An event may have a low probability of occurrence, but a high probability of serious consequences to patient and others, and this affects decision to investigate [399]

An investigation may be indicated to exclude a problem which could have implications for birth control or treatment of future illnesses [492]

The decisions in this case relate to diagnosis and the need for investigation (18).

The differential diagnosis includes a deep vein thrombosis and physical signs are unreliable in this condition. If there is a 1 in 10 probability of a deep vein thrombosis, should she be referred for investigation? Remember the facts in rule 399.

In all cases where thrombosis is suspected a careful history must be taken to identify factors that increase the risk. If she had recently flown home from Australia this would increase the risk of thrombosis. If she is not referred for investigation and later requests to be put on the contraceptive pill, would you agree or suggest another form of contraception? (492)

If this is a deep vein thrombosis it is the patient who is at risk of a pulmonary embolus and not the doctor. She has the right to be involved in any decision about investigation, treatment, or place of care. How could this be achieved? She could be told the following: "There is a possibility of a clot of blood in the deep veins of the leg. This cannot be excluded by examination alone. Although not very likely, if this is present, there is a small risk that it could pass into the lungs. This could be prevented by treatment to dissolve away the clot. The diagnosis can be confirmed by a test that can be done in hospital and would need to be organised as soon as possible. What do you feel about this?"

Such an approach does involve the patient. If the doctor does not mention the possibility of a deep vein thrombosis, the patient will be denied the right to share in an important management decision.

Case 22

A woman aged 53 was successfully operated on three years ago for carcinoma of bronchus. At outpatient follow up she was found to have a gland that, at biopsy, proved to be a high grade lymphoma. The surgeon says that she is fit and is reluctant to investigate further but will review her again in six months. You discuss the management options with the patient who then decided to be referred to the lymphoma clinic at the teaching hospital. Three months later she consults you in a worried and agitated state. She says that the slides sent from the hospital where the biopsy was done to the lymphoma clinic have been lost. She is therefore being admitted for thoracotomy and gland biopsy as mediastinoscopy was too difficult. She is very worried but prepared to have this done. "Have I made the right decision doctor?"

> If investigation results are lost, they may sometimes be duplicated or repeated without involving the patient   [274]

The slides are needed to confirm the diagnosis and determine the most appropriate treatment. Unfortunately the slides have been lost and the patient faces a major invasive test. The GP may not seem to be the most appropriate person to deal with this problem; however, it is the cause of the presenting anxiety. How thorough was the search for these slides? This was discussed with the clinic registrar who said that they had looked everywhere they could think of. He had also checked that they had been posted (274).

> If slides are lost, new ones may be made without repeating the biopsy investigation as the original material is kept for some years   [442]

Can a duplication of the results be done for this patient? (442) A telephone call to the hospital pathologist confirmed that it would be easy to duplicate the lost slides. This was done and the patient avoided a thoracotomy. It was difficult to understand why this option was never considered. Patients often find a second opinion from their GP of value.

Case 23

A woman aged 58 had a breast carcinoma removed three years previously, and a local recurrence removed nine months previously. She had a routine bone scan done three weeks before which was normal. Today she came because she had coughed up some blood. She thinks, however, that it may have come from the nose. On examination the chest is clear and no blood is seen in the throat or nose. She now feels well, even though it only occurred that morning. What is your management?

> The patient's explanation or diagnosis of a problem is always significant, but does not outweigh a good differential diagnosis   [457]

This is a diagnostic problem (457).

In making a diagnosis it is important to decide if two observations or events are related or coincidental [115]

A chest radiograph was done which was normal. Before deciding not to undertake further investigations all the relevant factors must be considered (115).

If she was a smoker would this influence the decision to refer her for bronchoscopy? There is no objective evidence of cancer, and she stopped smoking 18 months ago. What is the probability of cancer in a past smoker who has recently coughed up a small amount of blood, but who has a normal chest radiograph? The decision about the need for further investigations should be shared with the patient. What would you do if there was a 5% risk of a carcinoma of the bronchus in such cases? One option is to say that at present further tests are not needed, but if more blood is coughed up further investigations should be done. This approach ignores the right of the patient to share the decision. Consider the following explanation:

> You have coughed up some blood and it is reassuring that the X-ray was normal. However, you were a smoker until recently and there is a small possibility that there could be a growth that does not show on the X-ray. (Perhaps a 5% chance.) A bronchoscopy is the only definite way to exclude this less common but more serious cause of coughing up blood. This involves an anaesthetic and examination of the airways by passing a tube into them. If a growth was too small to be seen on the X-ray but was found on bronchoscopy, there is a good chance of surgical removal.

This explanation could enable the patient to share in this critically important decision. In this case she decided to have the bronchoscopy. A small operable carcinoma was found and she made a good long-term recovery.

Case 24

A woman aged 65 was seen in evening surgery. She had had haematuria for four days without pain or fever. Two years ago she had had an atrial flutter and was put on long term warfarin to prevent emboli. The arrhythmia has been well controlled on digoxin and quinidine. She has been discharged from the cardiac clinic. There were no abnormalities on abdominal, vaginal, or rectal examination. The urine contained microscopic haematuria. What is your management?

There are three differential diagnoses here. The haematuria could be the result of the warfarin. The other possibilities are that it is caused by an infection or growth. Is the haematuria related to her current treatment or the result of some other illness? When a differential diagnosis has been made, it is important to determine the order in which these ought to be excluded. The saying "the assumption that the most common things are the most likely" is responsible for many serious errors of judgement. It is more important to exclude less common but more serious conditions before more common but less serious ones. Potentially the most serious condition in terms of immediate risk would be bleeding caused by warfarin (32).

The anticoagulant control of this patient is the first thing that needs checking. Should a prothrombin time be done if she was seen at 7 p.m. or can it wait until the morning? Much will depend on the risks that you are prepared to take. Are there other signs of haemorrhage such as bruising or petechiae? If her prothrombin time were dangerously high, she would need treatment tonight (482).

The hospital will do out of hours tests if indicated. Her prothrombin time was within an acceptable range. A midstream urine specimen was sterile and an ultrasonogram was normal. She could be asked to return if there is any recurrence of blood in the urine, or she could be referred for further investigations. There is still a possibility of malignancy and this cannot be excluded without cystoscopy. She is taking warfarin, which might be contraindicated in the presence of a growth that could bleed. Is this a decision you feel able to take or should it be shared with the patient or hospital consultant? (261)

How would you explain the options to this woman? Mentioning cancer might cause considerable anxiety. Is this a sufficiently good reason for not involving the patient in this decision? If you feel strongly that referral is indicated, you may advise the patient that further investigations are needed to exclude serious disease. If you feel equivocal about referral, however, the patient could be allowed

> The management of a woman with haematuria and dysuria is different if investigations have excluded either drug side effects, for example, warfarin or a urinary tract infection [32]

> Investigations should be done urgently if there is a probability of a disease for which immediate admission, treatment, or isolation would be indicated [482]

> The doctor must constantly ask whose decision this is to safeguard the rights of the patient [261]

> "Most common causes have been excluded. There is a small possibility that there could be a small growth in the bladder. Although this is a small risk, it cannot be excluded without a test involving an examination of the bladder. Would you like to have this done, or would you prefer to consider this if there is any recurrence of bleeding?"

> GPs must reassess indications for long term therapy if this was started by the hospital and the patient was subsequently discharged from follow up [480]

to decide. It may be reasonable to give the advice in the box.

Patients sometimes ask their GP to decide for them. This is perfectly acceptable but at least they have been given the chance to be involved. This patient decided to undergo cystoscopy which proved normal. She needs to know what to do if the bleeding recurs.

Does she still need to be on warfarin? Five years ago, when she was discharged from hospital, it was thought that she should continue this drug. Indications for long term treatment do, however, change over time (480).

If a patient has been discharged from hospital on long term therapy, it is the GP's responsibility to ensure that it is still indicated. In this case, the cardiologist was telephoned and he suggested that the warfarin could be stopped safely. Many patients are discharged from hospital on warfarin and attend the anticoagulant clinic. In the absence of clear guidelines from the hospital consultant, the GP is responsible for decisions about the need for long term therapy. The discharge summary should have indicated for how long the warfarin should be continued. This does not always happen.

Case 25

A woman aged 38, married with two daughters, requests a test for Huntington's disease. She has a family history of early dementia in both her mother and her grandmother. She is taking out a life insurance policy and the company asked her to have a test for this genetic disease. She had a depressive illness five years ago which was successfully treated with no recurrence. There is no other significant history. What is your management?

Anyone offered a test for a
genetic disease must understand
that it is voluntary and be told:

● about the disease he or she
may have

● what can be done to treat it

● how reliable the test is

● how a positive result might
affect his or her family[1]   [897]

She has been asked to have a test which, if positive, could have profound effects on her and others in the family. She needs to be counselled before having such a test, and the GP must decide who should undertake this task (897).

Informed consent is needed before doing this test. This patient was referred to a clinical geneticist who discussed the test's accuracy, benefits, risks, emotional and social sequelae, and treatment options for the disease.

Case 26

A woman aged 26 with severe arthritis comes to see you complaining of weakness in her legs and hands for three weeks. You refer her urgently to the neurology clinic. Two weeks later the senior house officer telephones to say that she has signs of spasticity in all limbs and they suspect early onset of spastic quadriplegia caused by cord compression in the neck. She needs an urgent MRI scan but the hospital has spent all its allocated budget for this investigation and there is no money to do this test. He says that the consultant has discussed the case with the director of the radiology department who says that she cannot authorise this scan because they have only been funded for a specific number by the purchasing authority, and these have all been done. He asks if you are a fund holder but you are not. He says that he does not know what more can be done and asks for your suggestions. What is your response?

● Talking to the consultant
neurologist

● Talking to the radiologist

● Suggesting that the hospital
staff deal with this problem

● Discussing the issue with the
purchasers

● Considering an extra
contractual referral

● Talking to the chief executive

It is surprising that this problem is presented to the GP. It is even more amazing that this task has been delegated to the senior house officer. I could hardly believe my ears. Options include those shown in the box.

Consultants, managers, purchasers, and providers are all responsible for trying to resolve problems that arise when patients need urgent investigations or treatments, and budgets have been spent

[686]

This problem seems to be about shortage of resources or inadequate budgets. It is also about failure to identify whose responsibility this is. Should it be the director of the medical or radiology departments, the hospital managers, the purchasers, or a combination of these people? (686) There seems to be no policy for dealing with this problem. If one does exist, it is not being followed. The delegation of this telephone call to one of the most junior doctors in the team indicates poor judgement. The consultants do not seem to know how to handle this problem. The extra contractual referral procedure was not set up to let the hospital off the hook in these situations.

The senior house officer was assured that this was not her problem. She was told that a way would be found to sort it out and that the hospital would be contacted later that morning. There did not seem much point in discussing this with the consultants. The manager responsible for purchasing radiology services from this hospital was immediately contacted. He gave an assurance that there were contingency funds for such situations, and that he was very surprised that the hospital managers had not dealt with this problem. He was asked to educate the hospital consultants and managers in the correct procedures to follow should such a problem recur. He was also asked to telephone back to say what had been organised. He telephoned back an hour later to say that everything had been dealt with. Patients should never be involved in such mismanagement.

After decisions have been made about diagnosis and investigations, doctors and their patients must select appropriate management objectives. Measuring the effectiveness of treatment is made easier when measurable goals have been identified.

Conclusion

Decisions about investigations depend on your perception of the problem. The single most important suggestion is therefore to listen to patients without any interruption

until they have finished talking. This gives the best opportunity to identify the nature of the problem and the
need for further clarification.

1 *Genetic Screening, Ethical Issues*, 1993. Available from Nuffield Council
on Bioethics, 28 Bedford Square, London WC1B 3EG.

10 Objectives

- Prevent problems (primary prevention)
- Treat and prevent disability, that is, cure (secondary prevention)
- Prevent deterioration or death in an incurable condition (tertiary prevention)

Decisions about the goals of treatment should be taken before the selection of the most appropriate management options. The goals involve primary, secondary, and tertiary prevention (see box).

In most consultations, primary prevention occurs alongside other goals such as treatment of the acute condition. In patients with chronic diseases who develop an acute illness, secondary and tertiary prevention are relevant objectives, because the acute condition may well cause a deterioration in the chronic illness. In such patients primary prevention may also be relevant for example, influenza immunisation.

Patients with a repeat prescription card for long term medication need regular follow ups to assess whether:

- management is still effective
- treatment is still being taken
- indications for treatment have changed
- all the drugs are still needed
- dosages are appropriate
- side effects have occurred
- drug interactions are likely
- problem list contains a new condition which may contraindicate a long term drug or be caused by it
- blood tests are needed
- new illness has developed that may require drug dosages to be changed
- a different form of treatment, for example, surgical is now indicated   [506]

Case 27

A man aged 56 with hypertension is on bendrofluazide and propranolol. He comes for a blood pressure check, because the repeat prescription card indicates that it is time for a review. The blood pressure is 190/130. He has no headaches and feels well. There are no signs of cardiac failure, and the urine and fundi are normal. What is your management?

What are the management objectives of such a consultation? (506)

Management objectives include assessing the need for, and the effectiveness of, treatment. A good opening question is "Are you still taking the tablets?" This implies a recognition that this may not be happening, and makes it easier for the patient to discuss this topic. The sequence of decision making is very important here (43).

Patients will often admit that they ran out of tablets a few days ago or are not taking the dose that has been prescribed. Changing the medication without assessing compliance creates a *folie à deux*. The patient may not be complying but does not like to say so. The doctor makes the wrong assumption and decides that the dose is inadequate. This rule describes the sequence in which decisions are made, that is, decide to do A before B. This patient ran out of tablets on Saturday and came to surgery on Monday. This was discovered by asking the above question. What questions might identify symptoms that could be the result of drug side effects in this patient? Enquiries should include impotence in men who are on β blockers long term.

> Assess compliance before changing medication or evaluating outcome or effectiveness   [43]

Case 28

A man aged 48 comes in with a cold. You notice a thyroidectomy scar from an operation for multinodular goitre 12 years before. He has no signs of hypothyroidism and feels fit. What is your management?

The management objectives in this case could be those in the box.

Management depends on having clear objectives. There will be several thyroidectomy patients in a practice of 12 000 patients. It is important for all the practice partners to agree on long term goals for this group of patients. It may be helpful to discuss this with the local endocrinologist before deciding what these should be (212).

> To prevent hypothyroidism
>
> To detect it before it produces symptoms
>
> To identify and treat it when symptoms appear

> It may be easier to prevent a disease than to diagnose it before it causes disability   [212]

A recall system is needed for safe follow up of patients:

- on long term medication
- who need periodic investigations or examinations
- who are on an at risk register   [194]

It is the patient's right to be given information on risk of surgical complications, both short and long term, and how these can be diagnosed or prevented   [411]

Hypothryoidism is difficult to diagnose clinically. Patients may be ill for many months before they seek advice for rather vague symptoms. If early detection is the goal, then decisions should be made about patients who should be screened, and how often this should be done (194).

Patients who have had thyroid surgery should be told of the risk of hypothyroidism, how this may be recognised, and what follow up is needed (411).

Unfortunately patients are rarely provided with this information. Early detection of hypothyroidism through annual screening of all patients below the age of 65 who have had thyroid surgery seemed an appropriate practice policy. Many patients need regular recall for examination or investigation. A practice recall register contains the name, diagnosis, need for recall, date, and outcome of recall. This is entered on a card or on the computer, so that patients who need thyroid tests can be identified opportunistically. The easiest time to do this is when a hospital letter is received stating that the patient has had a partial thyroidectomy or radioactive iodine treatment. The problem list should state that the patient is on the recall register.

Chronic disease management objectives

Clear objectives are needed for the management of chronic diseases. They are used to select appropriate treatment options and to audit the effectiveness of long term care. Below some examples are given for different chronic diseases.

Alcohol related problems

1. To control, reduce, or stop alcohol
2. To reduce level of intake (controlled drinking)
3. Identification and management of complications:
   - family
   - financial
   - legal
   - medical
   - neurological
   - nutritional
   - occupational
   - psychiatric
   - psychological
   - social
   - violence
4. Assessment of urgency, disability, severity, dependence
5. To reverse complications
6. To prevent complications
7. To prevent further deterioration
8. Restoration of normal function at home and work
9. Restoration of normal family relationships

Asthma

1. To prevent attacks
2. To treat attacks early and effectively
3. To prevent recurrent attacks
4. To prevent long term disability

Coronary artery disease

1. Prevention of disease
2. Identification of high risk groups
3. Alteration of lifestyle in high risk groups:
   - diet
   - exercise
   - smoking
   - weight
4. Rehabilitation:
   - physical
   - social
   - occupational
   - psychological
   - sexual
5. Prevention of recurrence

Cerebrovascular accidents

1. To assess:
   - bowels, bladder function
   - deafness
   - disability
   - language disorder
   - mental state
   - movement mobility
   - receptive dysphasia
   - home environment
     - —toilet, bathroom
     - —steps, stairs
     - —kitchen, chairs, bed
2. To prevent complications:
   - bed sores, heel sores
   - constipation
   - contractures
   - depression, distress
   - hypostatic pneumonia
   - incontinence, contractures
   - malnutrition
   - obesity
   - shoulder dislocation
3. To improve function
4. To prevent recurrence of CVA
5. To obtain relevant claims and allowances

Dementia in elderly people

1. To identify problem:
   - duration
   - impact on patient
   - severity
2. To exclude:
   - preventable causes
   - treatable causes
   - iatrogenic causes
3. To identify:
   - treatable causes
   - iatrogenic causes
4. To assess problem for carer and family
5. To identify other problems carer may have
6. To ensure that claims and allowances are obtained
7. To obtain respite care when needed

Diabetes

1. To maintain blood sugar and Hb_{A1} levels within satisfactory levels
2. To abolish symptoms
3. To prevent complications:
   - blindness and visual impairment
   - cerebrovascular disease
   - end stage renal failure
   - foot ulceration and limb amputation
   - hyperlipidaemia
   - hypertension
   - ischaemic heart disease
   - peripheral vascular disease
   - premature mortality
4. To educate patient and family about disease and its management by self care, self monitoring, and self treatment.
5. To clarify the roles and responsibilities of patient, GP, practice nurse, and the diabetic clinic
6. To maintain normal function
7. To identify and treat complications as early as possible
8. To prevent iatrogenic problems
9. To prevent influenza

Epilepsy
1. To prevent:
   - disability
   - fits
   - physical injury
2. To reduce:
   - disability
   - risk of injury during fit
   - risk of injury to others
3. To treat fits promptly and effectively
4. To identify:
   - drug interactions
   - side effects
   - psychosocial problems
5. To provide long term follow up and evaluation
6. To educate patient and family
7. To advise about driving regulations and review

Mental illness
(including behavioural and psychological problems
1. To prevent illness
2. To prevent crises
3. To prevent relapse or recurrence
4. To prevent disability
5. To prevent self injury
6. To prevent psychological problems in family
7. Early treatment and crisis intervention
8. To maintain function:
   - social
   - occupational
   - daily living
9. To identify and treat side effects
10. Family assessment and support

Multiple sclerosis
1. To establish diagnosis
2. To assess disability at home and work
3. To prevent further disability
4. To maintain or improve function
5. To prevent complications:
   - bed sores
   - incontinence
   - muscle spasm
   - pain
6. To treat acute relapses
7. To maximise function

The objectives in the lists help to decide what the aims of treatment are, and clarify what the possible goals might be. Decisions about which management objectives to select should be shared with patients.

11 Management options

Management selection in patients with chronic illnesses depends on assessment of needs, clearly defined objectives, and knowledge of available options. Option "menus" can make selection decisions more appropriate and comprehensive. Management may sometimes be less effective because relevant options are not considered. Decision support, in the form of option menus for 25 conditions, has been developed and updated for use by trainees in our practice over many years. They have been found to be of great value to trainees who commented that they reduced management uncertainty. These option lists are not found in any textbook. Many options may be relevant for an individual patient. A few examples of option menus for some common conditions are listed below.

Asthma
1. To treat acute attack:
   - bronchodilators
     —oral inhalers
     —nebulisers
     —injections
     —suppositories
     —volumatic
   - steroids
     —inhalers
     —tablets
     —intravenous treatment
   - admit to hospital
2. Education:
   - monitoring disease
   - peak flow measurement and recording
   - symptom scores
   - house dust control
   - when to adjust treatment
   - when to start oral steroids
   - purpose of different medications
   - when to seek help
   - stop smoking
   - correct inhaler technique
3. To prevent recurrence:
   - antiallergic drugs
   - anti-inflammatory drugs
   - dust control
   - avoidance of precipitating factors
4. Influenza immunisation
5. To refer to:
   - chest physician
   - allergy clinic
   - general physician
   - nurse run asthma clinic
   - relaxation classes
   - allergy clinic
6. Self help groups
7. To investigate:
   - sputum tests
   - radiograph
   - sensitivity tests
   - peak flow readings
   - lung function tests
   - exclude iatrogenic causes, for example, β blockers
8. To put on disease register
9. To prescribe peak flowmeter and instruct on use
10. To modify smoking behaviour
11. To prescribe oral steroids and instructions for self medication
12. To enter on recall register for follow up
13. Written protocol on self management
14. To refer to National Asthma Campaign

Asthma—*continued*

15. To consider asthma when prescribing for other conditions
16. To consider drug interactions
17. To develop practice policy, for example, follow guidelines from British Thoracic Society
18. To follow up after recovery:
    - avoidable cause?
    - earlier call for help?
    - self medication appropriate?
    - peak flowmeter used and management adjusted?
19. To adjust long term medication
20. To develop a shared care scheme with hospital consultants

Mental illness

1. To assess problem:
   - mental, social, occupational, sexual, behavioural, in patient and family
   - severity and urgency
   - risk of self injury or violence
2. To assess needs of others including children
3. To provide family support
4. Counselling services
5. Drug therapy
6. To organise supervision of drug therapy
7. To monitor drug levels
8. To observe patient at risk
9. Support from relatives, neighbours
10. Behavioural therapy
11. Family therapy
12. To put on disease register for long term follow-up
13. To refer to:
    - community psychiatric nurse
    - psychologist
    - psychiatrist
    - counsellor
    - psychotherapist
    - behavioural nurse therapist
    - Relate
    - social worker
    - psychosexual clinic
    - emergency psychiatric clinic
    - drop in centres
    - local voluntary agencies (MIND, SANE)
    - psychiatric intervention team
    - psychiatric registrar in accident and emergency department
    - patient support groups
14. Psychiatric crisis intervention team assessment
15. Domiciliary psychiatric visit
16. Admission:
    - voluntary
    - section
17. Police assistance
18. Court injunction
19. Take children into care
20. Case conference
21. Follow up assessment
22. Blood tests:
    - drug levels
    - monitor thyroid function
23. To put on recall register
24. To initiate shared care record
25. To obtain claims and allowances, for example, disability benefit
26. Voluntary carers
27. Voluntary organisations SANE, MIND, Schizophrenia Fellowship, etc
28. Community follow up by key worker
29. To put on register of patients at risk of violent behaviour
30. Six to 12 months off driving after acute psychotic episode requiring hospital admission
31. Licence restored if:
    - free from symptoms in this period
    - demonstrates good compliance with medication
    - shows insight into condition
32. To identify patients who are on a community supervision order
33. To recommend relevant literature

Multiple sclerosis

1. To educate patient and family about illness and management
2. To assess needs
3. To refer to:
   - chiropodist
   - community care assessment
   - district rehabilitation officer
   - neurologist
   - occupational therapist
   - physiotherapist
   - psychologist
   - psychosexual counsellor
   - self help group
   - social worker
   - speech and language therapist
   - urologist
4. To order aids
5. Environmental control systems for severely disabled
6. Claims and allowances
7. Voluntary organisations
   - Multiple Sclerosis Society
   - SPOD (sexual/personal relationships of disabled)
8. Employment:
   - register disabled
   - refer to district rehabilitation officer
9. To refer for driving ability and car adaptation assessment
10. Community services:
    - meals on wheels, home care assistant
    - day care facilities, incontinence laundry services, bath attendant
11. Transport services:
    - dial a ride
    - orange badge
12. Domiciliary visit
13. Admit to:
    - district hospital
    - rehabilitation unit
14. Drugs:
    - ACTH, oral steroids
    - antispasmodics
    - carbamazepine
    - ephedrine
    - immunosuppressants
15. Admit to home for long term disabled
16. To consider residential homes
17. Dietary advice, prevent obesity
18. Respite care
19. Holidays for the disabled
20. Involve voluntary carers
21. Intermittent self catheterisation
22. Visit to Disabled Living Foundation
23. To give patient reference information in book[1]
24. To inform Driver and Vehicle Licensing Agency (DVLA)

Diabetes

1. To investigate:
   - confirm diagnosis
   —random blood sugar
   —glucose tolerance test (WHO criteria)
   - urine for ketones
2. To examine for indications for admission:
   - vomiting, dehydration
   - ketones in urine
   - severe infection
3. To educate patient:
   - practice information pack to standardise instructions and education
   - nurse or nurse practitioner
   - British Diabetic Association Handbook
4. To discuss management with patient and partner
5. Diet alone
6. Diet and tablets
7. To refer to:
   - dietician
   - diabetic clinic
   - diabetic liaison sister
   - district nurse
   - chiropodist
   - diabetic day care centre
8. Hospital admission
9. Shared care book
10. Disease register
11. To follow practice protocol
12. To allocate responsibility for education and its evaluation and follow up
13. To set up practice diabetic audit
14. To ensure trainees follow diabetic protocol
15. Recall scheme
16. To follow protocols for general practice management:
    - British Diabetic Association
    - local shared care protocol
    - practice protocol
17. To advise about:
    - exemption from prescription charges
    - informing DVLA
    - occupational implications

Conclusion

Option menus are derived from many different sources. I have developed these for 25 different chronic problems. They have been found to be a very useful decision aid for trainees and also for experienced doctors. They include a wide range of social, psychological, and medical options which are not found in any one book. Decisions about selection depend on current indications for specific forms of treatment. They need to be revised and updated from time to time. Before deciding on the most appropriate management, it is helpful to have a checklist of all possible options to ensure that some relevant strategies are not overlooked. Such lists are intended to be brief and comprehensive, but are difficult to remember. They make it easier to select most appropriate options for any individual patient at a specific point in time.

1 Burnfield A. *Multiple sclerosis: a personal exploration.* Condor book, Souvenir Press (E and A), 1985.

12 Indications

Health care is expensive and there should be good indications for the treatments selected. There should be clear criteria for certain forms of care, or treatment, based on evidence from randomised controlled trials. Sometimes such evidence is not available and indications may be based on expert opinion or consensus guidelines.

Case 29

A woman aged 51 presents with headaches for the last two months. There is a threat of redundancy and much stress at work. She is found to have a blood pressure of 185/120 but the fundi and urine are normal. An electrocardiogram and chest radiograph are also normal. What is your management? Would you treat this patient's hypertension or not? (164)

> One random observation may not be sufficient indication for starting long term treatment [164]

Hypertension is a condition that should not be diagnosed on the basis of one blood pressure reading alone. Treatment may be indicated on the basis of one reading if signs of end organ damage are present. These are absent in this patient (163).

This patient has two problems which may be related. She has considerable anxiety about the possibility of redundancy, and she also has a raised blood pressure. Her anxieties and fears should be explored, and the blood pressure should be taken again on three separate occasions before deciding whether treatment is needed. There ought to be a practice policy on indications for treating hypertension. Do all the doctors and nurses use the same diastolic end point? This is particularly important when many people are involved in screening and assessing effectiveness of therapy. Guidelines are updated periodically and they provide clear indications for levels at which treatment should be started.[1] They could form the basis for a practice protocol.

> The diagnosis of some problems necessitates several observations made at different times [163]

Case 30

A woman aged 29 is 32 weeks' pregnant. Antenatal care is being shared with the hospital. She has had some spotting of blood for the last two days. You refer her immediately to the obstetric registrar with the expectation that she will have a scan. A week later she comes back to surgery and says that she feels well. There has been no further bleeding and she says that a scan was not done. On routine antenatal examination everything is normal. A week later you visit because she has severe abdominal pain and a hard uterus. You diagnose a concealed antepartum haemorrhage and admit her to hospital. The baby is stillborn. The case management is being reviewed. Could the GP have managed this patient more effectively?

In such cases every effort should be made to identify preventable factors (563).

If ultrasonography had been done when she was initially referred, it might have shown something that may have needed urgent admission. In retrospect it is difficult to understand why ultrasonography was not considered. Perhaps it would have been advisable to have discussed this again with the obstetric consultant when she was seen the following week (315).

The real responsibility for ensuring that this test was done rests, however, with the GP (267).

Presumably previous scans would have excluded a placenta previa. The indication for ultrasonography at this time is to exclude a haemorrhage or blood clot in the uterus (688).

In cases of unexpected death or stillbirth, recent patient management should be reviewed to identify preventable factors [563]

Shared care with GP, other members of the primary care team, and hospital staff includes discussion about potentially serious problems that arise [315]

If the patient is referred for a relevant test or investigation which is not done, the GP must reassess indications at follow up [267]

Management decisions about potentially serious problems arising during pregnancy ought to be discussed with hospital staff and midwives who are also involved in shared care [688]

Others who need to be informed about deaths and stillbirths may include doctors, nurses, health visitors, midwives, and appointment and transport staff, and records should indicate who has been told [630]

In cases of unexpected death or stillbirth, a home visit should be made to provide bereavement counselling, support, and to re-establish confidence [105]

Uncertainty about the need for an investigation should be resolved by discussions with the consultant. Who else needs to be told about this stillbirth? (630, 105)

A home visit provides a chance for the family to ask many questions about antenatal care and the cause of the stillbirth.

Case 31

A man aged 34 with HIV infection is offered zidovudine by the hospital registrar; however, he cannot actually provide it because the patient does not quite fit the current indications for prescribing a drug at a cost of £3000 per year. The patient was asked to write to his GP to see if she would be prepared to prescribe it; she refused saying that it was too expensive. This is the reason that he has changed his GP and come to see you. What is your response to his request for this drug?

It is unethical to offer a specific National Health Service treatment or investigation if the current indications for its use are not present [611]

This patient has been told that he does not fulfil the treatment criteria. The real issue is whether there is evidence that this drug would benefit him and whether he fulfils the indications for its use. This registrar is not prepared to stick to the agreed indications. He is suggesting that an effective treatment is being withheld because of its cost. This could involve great financial hardship to patients and their families who may struggle to raise the money for this drug or feel guilty at not being able to do so (611).

If the GP were to prescribe this drug he or she would appear to disagree with the current indications. The behaviour of this registrar will cause distress to many patients and their families, and will disrupt the doctor–patient relationship; the issue must therefore be resolved by discussion with the relevant consultant. The patient needs to understand that management is constantly being reviewed in the light of new evidence of effectiveness of treatment at different stages of the disease (438).

Discussion between GP and consultant may be the best way to overcome management or ethical problems and meet patient's needs [438]

The patient was offered a chance to discuss his management with the consultant who clarified the facts and reassured him that his management was appropriate.

- Valid and based on the best available evidence
- Reliable, relevant, and applicable
- Comprehensive, specific, flexible, and up to date

Treatment guidelines

It may be difficult to identify clear indications for certain kinds of treatment. Trials may not have been carried out, the evidence may be inconclusive, or the trials poorly designed. The next best thing is to identify guidelines for the most cost effective form of treatment. Such guidelines or protocols do a great deal to ensure high quality care.[2] They should be based on the boxed requirements.

Such guidelines may be national, regional, local, or practice specific. These are dealt with in more detail in chapter 30 on protocols.

Appropriateness

How appropriate is the treatment of patients we send to hospital? Is this a question that GPs should ask about their hospital colleagues? A study in the Trent region showed that coronary angiography and coronary artery bypass operations were performed for inappropriate or equivocal reasons in 50% of cases.[3] The same was true in the North-West Thames region for 60% of cholecystectomies, regardless of whether they were performed in the public or the private sector.[4] Brook suggests that appropriateness ratings could revolutionise health care. Purchasers could decide to buy services only from doctors who agreed to provide services that satisfied generally accepted criteria of appropriateness. Ratings could also be used to prevent the underuse of necessary care. Brook has shown how such ratings can be made, and how the doctor and patient can use this information to plan present and future treatment.[5]

This has important implications for referral decisions by GPs. We need to know whether appropriate treatment is being purchased and provided for our patients. This information is important in decisions about care of individual patients, and should inform our dialogue with purchasers. Patients need to be reassured that, before they are subjected to a procedure or denied its use, its appropriateness has been explicitly verified. Methods to assess appropriateness are now available. It is time they were used by doctors and purchasers to eliminate both underuse and overuse of clinical interventions.

1 Summary of 1933 World Health Organization International Society of Hypertension guidelines for the management of mild hypertension. *BMJ* 1993;**308**:1541–6.

2 Grol R. Development of guidelines for general practice care. *Br J Gen Pract* 1993;**43**:146–51.

3 Gray D, Hampton JR, Bernstein SJ, Kosecoff J, Brook RH. Clinical practice: audit of coronary angiography and bypass surgery. *Lancet* 1990;**335**:1317–20.

4 Scott EA, Black N. Appropriateness of cholecystectomy: the public and private sectors compared. *Ann R Coll Surg Engl* 1992;**72**(suppl 4): 97–101.

5 Brook RH. Appropriateness: the next frontier. *BMJ* 1994;**308**:218–19.

13 Follow up and outcomes

The need for follow up is often overlooked. If the outcome of treatment needs to be assessed, then follow up is needed. The outcomes of care often depend on decisions about the need for follow up and the way this is organised.

Case 32

A boy aged 12 is visited by a deputising doctor at 1 a.m. Saturday. A note given to the parents is brought in by the father. It states that he has epididymo-orchitis and was given amoxycillin and co-proxamol. Father says that his pain is now less. There is no request for a visit. What is your management?

- Doing nothing more at this time
- Asking father to call if pain gets worse
- Telling him to telephone for a visit if pain is still present in 24 hours
- Asking him to bring the boy to the surgery immediately for reassessment
- Doing a home visit that morning
- Asking if he would like a home visit

Decisions that are made at this time will depend on the perception of the problem. Is it a diagnostic problem or does it relate to follow up? There is a great temptation to accept another doctor's diagnosis without considering other possibilities. Management options include those in the box.

Effective management depends on having clear goals and making the right decisions in the correct order. Appropriate management of this patient depends on an accurate differential diagnosis. The need for follow up reassessment will depend on the severity and urgency of the condition (1, 3, 4, 6).

Management of night visits by deputising service must be reviewed to decide if urgent follow up is needed   [1]

84

A follow up visit is indicated if deputising doctor's diagnosis could have included a potentially serious condition [3]

The differential diagnosis must always include conditions that may need surgical assessment [4]

If there is no obvious cause for swelling and pain in the testicle, admit to exclude torsion [6]

The decision to follow up or evaluate the outcome of a potentially serious problem is the responsibility of the doctor and not the patient [5]

The rules shown here present a loose sequence in which decisions need to be made. They also describe the factors that need to be considered and show how these might affect management decisions. Who should decide whether or not a follow up visit ought to be done? (5)

The decision to visit is based on professional judgement and should not be delegated to a relative. A visit was made immediately, and the boy was admitted and successfully operated on later that morning.

Case 33

A man aged 53 has pain and a palpable swelling in the right lower abdomen. Appendicitis is suspected and he is referred to hospital. He returns four days later, says that it was not appendicitis, and he now feels well. He wants a certificate to return to work. What do you do?

At follow up objective observations must be reassessed as well as subjective ones [7]

This seems a straightforward case. He wants a certificate to return to work. It was not appendicitis and he feels well. What more needs to be done? A certificate was given but should he have been re-examined? (7)

The patient was not re-examined and at the initial consultation there was a swelling as well as pain. Management would have been different if the swelling was still present. A decision that is often omitted is whether or not to re-examine a patient who had an abnormal finding, was referred to hospital, and subsequently discharged. Assumptions are no substitute for re-examination to ensure that abnormal findings have gone. This patient was sent to hospital with a suspected surgical condition (477).

Patients sent for admission by the GP but not admitted need follow up by the GP the next day [477]

Such patients should be told that if they are not admitted and the pain persists, they ought to be seen in the surgery or at home the following day.

Case 34

A woman aged 60 feels unwell. Your practice partner could not find any abnormality and agreed to her request for a private medical referral. The physician found a growth in the colon and referred her privately to a surgeon. He said that it was likely to be cancer and, although it could be done on the NHS, it is urgent and there was a waiting list. They decided to have it done privately. The operation was a success but the husband is now very worried because the cost will use up most of his savings. "What can I do about this doctor?"

A GP must clarify whether the objective of a private referral is only diagnostic, or whether it also includes private treatment

[54]

Assessment of patient's ability to pay should precede the decision to select private treatment   [17]

The GP lost control of this patient. What was the objective of this referral: for diagnosis only or also for private treatment? This must always be discussed with the patient who may not be aware of this critical distinction (54).

Many patients can afford a private consultation, but few can afford expensive investigations or treatment. It is essential that the goals are clearly specified in the referral letter (17).

This factor of cost will also determine the objectives of the private referral. If this had been clearly stated the patient would not have had to pay for private surgery. The correct procedure would have been to ask the consultant to assess the problem and to suggest the most appropriate treatment. The GP could then review the options, with reference to the waiting times, with the patient. This would precede any consideration of private treatment (15).

A patient sent as a private referral by a GP to a consultant ought to be sent back to the GP and not referred on to another private consultant   [15]

Private referrals should still be followed up to ensure that management is appropriate and cost effective   [36]

The patient needs to know what the objectives of the referral are. A follow up appointment should always be made to discuss the consultant's opinion with the patient. This enables treatment options to be reviewed (36).

This particular financial hardship could have been discussed with the consultant, in addition to the waiting times for cancer surgery. The advantage of a letter rather than a telephone call at this stage is that it gives the consultant time to formulate a more considered response. A letter was written stating what the patient "seemed to have understood" about the waiting list for people with possible malignancy and asking for clarification. It was pointed out that this had influenced the decision to have private treatment and the absence of insurance has caused severe financial hardship. The surgeon telephoned back to say that NHS treatment was offered but that it might take six weeks to get a bed. She had wanted him to do the operation but he explained that, under the NHS, he could not promise that he would be doing her operation. She opted for private treatment because she very much wanted him to do the operation. In view of the misunderstandings and the financial hardship he agreed to a substantial reduction in fees.

Case 35

A woman aged 45 is a mild asthmatic under the care of the chest clinic. She is on salbutamol, beclomethasone, and prednisolone 10 mg on alternate days. She comes for more tablets. The last letter from the consultant six weeks previously says that she remains well on the current dosage and is now being discharged from the clinic. She says she will be happy to see the patient again if any problems arise. The patient asks for a repeat prescription card. What is your management at this time?

Decisions about long term steroids are now your responsibility. All patients with repeat prescription cards for long term medication need regular follow up (506).

The objective is to find the lowest dose that will control her symptoms, and this will change over time. In fact many patients monitor their own illness (595).

After a patient with a chronic illness is discharged from hospital follow up, it is important to decide how long term care is to be organised. Is responsibility to be shared

---

Patients with a repeat prescription card for long term medication need regular follow up to assess whether:

- management is still effective
- treatment is still being taken
- indications for treatment have changed
- all the drugs are still needed
- dosages are appropriate
- side effects have occurred
- drug interactions are likely
- problem list contains a new condition which may contraindicate a long term drug or be caused by it
- blood tests are needed
- new illness has developed that may require drug dosages to be changed
- a different form of treatment is now indicated   [506]

Responsibility for management of a chronic illness should be shared with the patient who needs to be taught how to evaluate and adjust treatment, prevent relapses and complications, and take appropriate action when these occur   [595]

between the GP and the patient? If so, the education, skills, knowledge, and resources that both need must be identified:

- Does she have a peak flow machine?

- Is it used correctly?

- Are the results recorded accurately?

- Does she have written instructions on what to do when peak flows or symptoms change?

- Does she carry a steroid card?

- Has she been put on the disease register for follow up?

After discharge from hospital follow up there needs to be a reappraisal of the patient's knowledge skills and responsibilities. The patient also needs to know what responsibilities are the GP's. Is the management objective to find the lowest maintenance dose of steroids or try slowly to wean her off them completely? It could be useful to clarify this with the consultant.

Case 36

A man aged 67 comes to surgery with a skin problem. He has recently been to the skin clinic and the last two letters from the hospital are about this problem. You see that nine months ago he was seen by a urologist who says that clinically he has a carcinoma of prostate and needs to come in for biopsy. The patient says that he was sent for but no bed was available. Since that time he has not heard from the hospital. His last three visits to the surgery were for the skin problem and he was seen by a different doctor each time. What are the thoughts on this patient's management so far?

The objectives of the consultation are to:

- identify and manage acute illness
- review management of coexisting chronic illness
- screen for health problems and risk factors and prevent or treat as necessary
- modify future help seeking behaviour where appropriate

[375]

This case highlights the difficulty of remembering to manage coexisting problems at the same time as the presenting complaint. This needs to be built into a routine task at every consultation (375).

In a group practice where continuity of care is not always possible, fail safe procedures are needed to ensure effective follow up of potentially serious problems [346]

Patients with a potentially serious problem who are put on waiting list for further investigations or treatment should:

- have this entered on their problem list
- be recalled for follow up within a definite period of time to find out if tests or treatment have been done [345]

Identification of the cause of mistakes is as important as making a differential diagnosis of an observation or symptom [756]

The aetiology of a serious administrative or clerical error must be identified to prevent recurrence [350]

Two things happened in this case: the hospital failed to recall him and the GPs failed to notice the preceding problem (346).

How could effective follow up be done? The time to take action is on receipt of the hospital letter (345).

"Fail safe" mechanisms are needed to prevent this sort of problem. Patients must not endure waiting periods that could affect their life expectancy. There should be a practice policy about such patients; two options could be considered. When a hospital letter is received saying malignancy is suspected, this information could be entered on the problem list. The other option is to complete a recall card for the patient. This contains name, date of birth, date of recall, and is filed by month. This would enable the receptionist to pull the notes and check if there is any information about follow up investigations. If not, the GP can telephone the patient or contact the hospital to find out what has happened. What should be done for this patient now? It looks as if an organisational error has resulted in him being overlooked, but there might be other explanations (756).

The initial reaction is to assume that the hospital has overlooked this patient (350). If there is a letter in the notes saying that he had not attended for further tests, the GP would have to accept some responsibility for this delay. Perhaps the patient has moved and not informed the hospital of his new address?

There are two management objectives: one is to get him investigated and treated as soon as possible; the other relates to prevention of recurrence. In this situation it is always best to telephone and discuss the problem with the consultant. Remember that there are two things to discuss: the first is when to admit and the second relates to a tighter follow up procedure. This should be applied by the GP as well as by the hospital staff.

Case 37

A man aged 55 is discharged from hospital after having a haematemesis caused by a duodenal ulcer. He has been given a seven day supply of ranitidine, but was not told of any need to continue taking this medication.

He returns to see you a month later to request a repeat prescription for his regular drugs. It said "see doctor" on his repeat prescription card and he has to see the GP before he can be given another supply of naproxen which he takes for mild ankylosing spondylitis. What is your management?

> Long term medication must be reviewed after hospital discharge to ensure that it is not contraindicated by the new illness [730]

How do you see this problem? Why is this a potentially dangerous situation? (730)

> Patients discharged on hospital drugs need to distinguish between short and long term medication [728]

This patient has restarted the arthritis treatment he was taking before his admission to hospital. Is this appropriate? (728)

> ● Old diseases–new disease
> ● Old treatments–new treatments
> ● Old treatments–new disease
> ● New treatments–old diseases

The interactions that must be considered in patients who have been discharged from hospital include those between the pairs in the box. In this case the important interactions are between old treatments and new disease (730).

> Long term medication must be reviewed after hospital discharge to ensure that it is not contraindicated by the new illness [730]

This patient's perforation could have resulted from the naproxen; non-steroidal drugs would therefore be contraindicated in this patient from now on. This was not identified as a problem in the hospital discharge letter. He was admitted as an emergency by the deputising doctor and the hospital staff may not have known about the long term naproxen treatment. Even if they had, not all hospital staff check whether it is safe to continue the long term medication being taken before admission (729).

> The practice must have a fail safe procedure to ensure that hospital medication on discharge is checked against any prior long term medication to ensure that:
> ● it is still needed
> ● there are no new contraindications
> ● it is compatible with the new medication [729]

How could this problem have been prevented? The receptionist could be asked to get out the records of patients when a discharge note is received from the hospital. Long term medication could then be reviewed alongside the drugs on discharge and the new illness.

Patients who did not attend

Many patients fail to attend the surgery or the outpatient clinic after appointments have been made. It is important to identify why a patient did not attend the outpatient clinic (639).

The practice should have a policy for dealing with the problem of non-attendance. The goals are to prevent serious problems being overlooked and to educate patients about the need to cancel if they cannot keep the appointment. It is difficult to remember the reasons for the referral. It would help if the hospital returned the referral letter with the note saying that the patient had not attended (10).

> The reasons patients default on their appointments or do not attend their hospital outpatient clinic include:
> - appointment not received
> - too ill to go
> - transport did not arrive
> - computer cancellation
> - problem resolved
>
> Follow up must clarify need for hospital referral [639]

> To prevent problems arising in defaulters and patients who did not attend, fail safe procedures must be developed [10]

Case 38

A woman aged 19 is four months' pregnant and many risk factors are present. She attended the practice antenatal clinic initially, but has not done so for the last four months. The hospital midwife phones to say that she has had an intrauterine death at eight months. The health visitor normally visits all defaulters but this time the health visitor was from another district. She did visit but was told by the patient that she was attending the hospital. This was not so. What is your management?

This is a high risk patient who was not followed up after defaulting from the antenatal clinic (133).

Who is responsible for such defaulting patients? (26)

This patient has defaulted from both the practice and hospital follow up. If such a patient was thought suitable for shared care, there must be clear lines of communication (562). This did not happen in this case. There has to be a fail safe routine to ensure communication occurs. Someone has to be responsible for reviewing the records of patients who did not attend the hospital or practice antenatal clinic. Some of these patients will be high risk

> Antenatal defaulters have a higher morbidity and perinatal mortality and need careful follow up [133]

> The GP is responsible for follow up of patients who default or did not attend, unless someone else has agreed to take on this task [26]

> Shared care means hospital staff and GP communicate when patient defaults from follow up [562]

91

- Which groups of defaulters need urgent follow up in the community?
- Who should be informed?
- Who should contact the patient?

High risk pregnant women who do not attend antenatal clinic may need follow up antenatal care at home   [714]

In cases of unexpected death, recent patient management should be reviewed to identify preventable factors   [563]

and other colleagues need to be informed. There should be a policy on the points in the box.

It may be appropriate to inform the midwife, health visitor, and GP. The task of ensuring that high risk defaulters are followed up should be delegated to a specific person, and everyone should know who this is. If someone else is asked to undertake such a follow up, the notes should record this delegation. The clinic is not the only place where antenatal care can be provided (714).

If shared care antenatal records are held by the patient, the health visitor should have asked to see them. This would have identified any problems and shown that the patient had not attended. Hospital staff change very frequently but in general practice the antenatal care tends to be provided by the same group of people. It may be easier for someone in the practice antenatal team to contact the hospital to find out what is happening to a high risk patient who has not been seen for some time. Perhaps the booking criteria were changed and she is now receiving total hospital care. Assumptions about the type of care being given are no substitute for facts. Could better communication have prevented the intrauterine death in this patient? (563)

When a death occurs, much can be learned from reviewing the management and organisation of care. If this was shared, the review should include everyone who was involved. The aim is not to allocate blame, but to see if a recurrence can be prevented by a change in the way the service is organised.

Case 39

A mother brings her child aged four years to Saturday morning surgery with a fever and rapid breathing. On examination of the chest there were no abnormal signs. She was referred to hospital with suspected pneumonia. At 4 p.m. the mother telephones to say that she has a right middle lobe pneumonia, but as she seemed better than she was in the morning she was thought to be suitable for home care. She has been given an antibiotic and seems comfortable. The mother was told to return to hospital if the child gets worse. What is your management now?

To provide effective home care and follow up, ill patients and their relatives need information about:

- what to do
- how to identify complications or deterioration
- what to do about them
- when to call the doctor
- what to do if no better within a specified period of time or if condition deteriorates
- when doctor will revisit

[472]

- Rapid or noisy breathing
- Movements of the nostrils in and out
- Temperature of over 103°F (39°C)
- Confusion or twitching
- Vomiting
- Fever lasting more than three days

When a hospital letter states that an appointment will be made it is the GP's responsibility to follow this up and ensure that it has been done   [82]

A GP referral letter may be indicated even if the patient was seen in the accident and emergency department and subsequently referred for an outpatient clinic appointment

[676]

This child is being given the correct treatment and it is obviously better to be at home than in hospital. Instructions have been given to return to the hospital if the child gets worse. But she has not been told what observations to make to identify deterioration (472).

This child has pneumonia. Instructions that would enable the mother to identify deterioration might include returning to hospital or seeing the GP if any of the signs in the box develop.

The mother may believe that all these observations must be present before she takes any action. Clear written instructions are essential to prevent complications when potentially serious conditions are treated at home.

The next decision relates to responsibility for follow up. If there is no deterioration, then this child will not be seen again in hospital and the GP is responsible for immediate follow up. She needs therefore to be told when to bring the child for review in the surgery. The next day a note is received from the accident and emergency department saying that she will be sent a follow up outpatient appointment (82).

It would be useful if hospital letters indicated whether an appointment has actually been sent. For "will be" read "maybe" as this is sometimes overlooked. This was the second episode of pneumonia that this child has had in 18 months. This past history may not be known to the outpatient doctor (676).

In this case a referral letter was sent saying that this was the second bout of pneumonia, and the father's past history of intravenous drug addiction was also mentioned.

Prevention of recurrence should always be considered, especially when the outcome of treatment is being assessed. The goal may be to prevent a recurrence, or to consider primary prevention, for example, influenza immunisation, in a patient with a chronic illness.

Conclusion

At the end of each consultation the GP should ask whether the patient needs to be seen again and, if so, why. Effective outcomes may well depend on remembering to ask these questions and making follow up decisions that are communicated clearly to the patient.

14 Prevention

Prevention is a task that has to be undertaken alongside the other objectives of the consultation. These include treatment of acute illness, management of coexisting chronic disease, and modification of help seeking behaviour.[1] In the UK, health promotion targets have been introduced and primary prevention has become an opportunistic component of each consultation. Prevention of recurrence or relapses is, however, also an important goal.

Case 39

An Asian mother brings her baby aged five months because the child has a cold. There is no fever and the chest is clear. There are no other abnormal findings. What is your management?

Management of the cold is the main concern for the mother but other management goals are also relevant (375).

What preventable medical condition should be considered in this baby? (107) There are two possible preventive goals for this child: one is the prevention of infectious diseases (109).

This goal should be considered when any child of this age is seen. The GP must, however, also be aware of the risks that different ethnic groups are exposed to.

The objectives of the consultation are to:

- identify and manage acute illness
- review management of coexisting chronic health problems
- screen for health problems and risk factors, and treat or prevent as needed
- modify future help seeking behaviour as appropriate

[375]

An important management objective is to prevent problems in at risk patients   [107]

An important management objective is to identify non-immunised children   [109]

An important management objective is to prevent osteomalacia in high risk groups [108]

The other goal is to prevent osteomalacia (108).

The key to prevention is to think in terms of risk. Is this patient at risk of developing a preventable disease? This child is at risk of osteomalacia which can be prevented by long term vitamin supplements. Effective preventive measures depend on opportunistic screening for risk factors which should become a routine part of every consultation.

Case 40

A woman aged 27 complains of a sore throat for one day. Seven months ago she had a quinsy which was drained in hospital. She has not seen a doctor since discharge as she has remained well. She now has pain on the same side of the throat as the quinsy. On examination she is afebrile, the tonsils look normal, but there is a slight swelling of the palate on one side. You suspect an early recurrence of quinsy. What is your management?

Unless otherwise stated in the hospital letter, responsibility for prevention of recurrence rests with the GP [589]

Follow up management of acute illness involves prevention of recurrence if possible [119]

To prevent a recurrence surgical referral may be necessary [425]

Management objectives should always include prevention of recurrence wherever feasible. This should be part of follow up management (589, 119).

Could this recurrence have been prevented? (425) Did the hospital discharge letter suggest referral to an ear, nose, and throat specialist? If the GP felt such a referral was indicated, why was this not arranged? The patient needs antibiotic treatment and daily follow up, and should be told to call or return earlier if symptoms get worse. The need for a specialist opinion needs to be discussed with the patient. A referrral should be made to decide whether a tonsillectomy is indicated to prevent recurrence of quinsy.

Case 41

A man aged 47 has had ulcerative colitis since he was 27. His colitis is well controlled and he is now fit. The disease affects the whole of the rectum and colon. Colonoscopies are carried out every year in view of the 15% risk of malignancy. He wants to know if it would be safer to have a colectomy to remove any risk of cancer developing. "What do you think, doctor?"

It is important to avoid the "if it were me" response. It is the patient's values and fears that are relevant and not those of the doctor. There are two options and both have risks. Annual colonoscopy has the risk that a growth may not be detected until it is too late for cure. Prophylactic surgery has a mortality risk and a risk of complications, but it removes the risk of cancer. The acceptability of a colostomy may need to be considered but some colectomy techniques can avoid the need for a colostomy (430).

> Patients need accurate information about effectiveness of screening versus risks, benefits, and disabilities of prophylactic surgery [430]

The GP's role is to help the patient to find the answers to the right sort of questions. A gastroenterologist would be the best person to provide this sort of information. The consultant was telephoned and agreed to discuss these issues with the patient. The patient should still take a referral letter to remind the consultant of the reason for the appointment.

Case 42

A woman aged 28 has three children aged seven, four, and two years. Her husband is a very successful barrister. He has decided to leave his wife and family to live with another woman. This is an irreversible decision on his part. His wife has come to see you for advice on how the news should be broken to the children. What are your suggestions?

One of the management objectives in this case is to reduce the psychological trauma to the children (483, 484). Sometimes parents do not recognise the trauma their behaviour can inflict.

> When relationships break down, communication between parents is essential to minimise psychological distress in children [483]

> The GP must ensure that both parents recognise the psychological effects their behaviour may have on the children [484]

The mother wants to reduce the psychological trauma this will cause the children. She wants to know the "what, when, how, and who" of telling the children. Do you feel competent to advise her at this time? (272)

> Children should be given information in a way that reduces psychological trauma and specialist advice may be needed on how best to do this [272]

To reduce psychological trauma of divorce or separation in very young children, parents should agree to say that the decision to separate is:

- mutual (no one parent to blame)
- irreversible (reduces guilt felt by children at failure of attempts to bring parents together again).

Also the parent who leaves will visit regularly [445]

After divorce or separation, follow up of young children is needed to assess adjustment and psychological state [446]

Parental separation or divorce should be entered on the children's problem lists as well as on those of both parents [447]

The skills needed to give this information to children are usually beyond the scope of the GP and specialist advice should be sought, as it is important to get this right. An appointment was made for both parents to see a child psychiatrist who made the suggestions in rule 445.

The mother found this advice very difficult as she had to accept part of the blame and guilt. She also had to tolerate her husband's presence three evenings a week initially, visiting and bathing the children. The psychiatrist thought that he should not take the children to meet his new partner at this time. His wife realised that this was a temporary measure of benefit to the children. Another objective is to follow these children up to identify and treat any behavioural or psychological problems that may arise (446).

In a group practice it is important for all doctors to know that there has been a parental separation. Another doctor seeing one of these children needs to know this family's background (447). The mother did not want to see a counsellor but was seen for brief support sessions of half an hour every two weeks for the next three months.

Another goal is to ensure that this patient has good legal representation. Her husband suggested that their family lawyer, who was also a friend, should act for them both. The GP suggested that she should be represented by a really tough woman lawyer.

Case 43

A man aged 52 has a past history of duodenal ulcer and myocardial infarction. He is a heavy smoker. He has remained well for the last two years. Now he complains of "palpitations" for the last three days, but no chest pain or dyspnoea. On examination there are occasional ectopic beats, but no other abnormalities. What is your management?

- Investigation by GP
- Referral to outpatient clinic
- Ask registrar to see today
- Allow to continue to work while awaiting appointment
- Do nothing but reassess in a week or earlier if palpitations recur

Investigations should be done urgently if there is a probability of a disease for which immediate admission, treatment, or isolation would be indicated [482]

To prevent coronary thrombosis or stroke, high risk patients should be given prophylactic treatment with low dose aspirin [719]

The decision about fitness for work pending investigation depends on:

- occupation
- risk to others and to patient if symptoms recur
- current disability
- natural history
- differential diagnosis
- risk of spread of infection
- risk and severity of complications
- legal requirements
- occupational guidelines
- past history [567]

The options include those in the box.

The differential diagnosis includes a recent coronary thrombosis (482). If facilities are available, should an electrocardiogram be done in the surgery? If it is normal, what should the management be? There are two objectives: one goal is to prevent another coronary thrombosis, the other to prevent further arrhythmias. The patient is still smoking, and this needs to be discussed.

Should he be taking any medication? (719) It would be appropriate to prescribe daily aspirin, and to ensure that he understands why this is needed. Is medication indicated for prevention of further arrhythmias or should he return if it recurs? This is a difficult decision to make and expert advice may help to clarify management. He could be referred to the medical registrar or the cardiology registrar could be asked to give an opinion. If it was decided to get an urgent appointment, what advice should be given about working? The need to make this decision is often over-looked (567).

What follow up is needed here? It may be advisable to ask the patient to return or call for a visit if the "palpitations" recur or if he develops pain or breathlessness.

An asthmatic attack can be precipitated by anxiety, stress, or psychological trauma the underlying aetiology of which needs to be identified, because successful management necessitates treatment of mental and physical state as well as prevention of recurrence   [520]

Long term medication may be necessary to prevent recurrence or relapse of certain diseases
[712]

A differential diagnosis must be made of treatment failure which includes factors related to diagnosis, natural history, presence of complications, patient's behaviour, information given, treatment, dosage, compliance, prevention of recurrence, coexisting diseases and their treatment, and follow up provided   [591]

Follow up management of acute illness involves prevention of recurrence if possible   [119]

Information given to patient should include how to prevent a recurrence and what to do if the problem recurs   [23]

Patients with a chronic disease who go on holiday need medication and instructions to prevent and treat relapse or complications   [717]

Case 44

An asthmatic woman aged 30 is now recovering from an acute attack which required steroids for control. Normally she is fit and only occasionally requires a salbutamol inhaler. She is going to Greece on holiday in four weeks and then on to the USA for a month. "Should I take any special precautions, doctor?" What is your response?

Were there any precipitating factors? (520)

After an acute attack, decisions need to be made about current medication (712).

What was she taking before this attack? Does the recent history suggest that she should have consulted the doctor earlier? (591)

After an acute attack compliance should be reviewed. The management objective now is to prevent recurrence (119). To achieve this the patient should be given clear written guidelines (23).

If she was not already taking beclomethasone, this preventive treatment should now be added to her current therapy. Does she monitor her own illness using a peak flowmeter, supported by written instructions on how to adjust her treatment? If not, would you provide this? What should she do if an attack does not respond to inhaler therapy? (717)

Effective emergency treatment
may be given by carers or
patient if informed about:

- what to look for and do
- what medication to take and
  when and how to take it
- what to do if no response or
  worse, or not better in
  specified period of time
- when to consult doctor   [429]

Instructions should contain a self management plan if
deterioration occurs (429). She should be given a course
of oral steroids and written instructions on when and how
to take them. She was also advised to take out a medical
insurance policy.

Case 45

A man aged 57 returns home after hospital treatment for
a coronary thrombosis. He weighs 22 stone and has made
a good recovery from his chest infection. While in hospital he developed severe back pain and was diagnosed as
having a prolapsed intervertebral disc. He has been lying
on the floor for two days and has asked you to visit
because he is no better and needs more analgesics. His
straight leg raising is limited to 30° but reflexes, sensation, and micturation are normal. What is your
management?

Which of the preventive goals in rule 64 are appropriate
for this patient? (64)

The objectives are to prevent coronary thrombosis and to
treat his prolapsed disc (599). The conventional management for a prolapsed disc would be to lie flat on a hard
surface. This can, however, increase the risk of thrombosis
(627).

Management decisions must be
related to one or more of the
following objectives:

- prevention of illness
- prevention of disability in
  curable illness
- prevention of further disability
  in chronic diseases
- prevention of recurrence or
  relapse
- prevention of death   [64]

The complications of some
treatments can be predicted and
prevented   [599]

Prediction of risk of serious
problems must always be
followed by appropriate
management to ensure its
prevention or early
identification   [627]

In general practice an important management objective is to identify patients at risk of deep vein thrombosis and take appropriate preventive action, for example, low dose heparin

[626]

There is a high risk of deep vein thrombosis in a 22 stone man who is immobilised and an important management objective is to prevent this complication (626). The risk of thrombosis was discussed and the patient agreed to take low dose heparin. These can be prescribed in syringes which most patients can be taught to self administer. They should dispose of the needles and syringes in a drinks can sealed with Sellotape.

The prevention of thrombosis in high risk groups is not considered as often as it should be. When patients develop an acute illness that causes immobility for any length of time, the risk of thrombosis should always be considered and a decision should be made about prevention with low dose heparin. This is a potentially life saving measure of proven effectiveness and minimal risk.

Case 46

A man aged 23 comes to say that he was assaulted and bitten by a complete stranger in the street two days previously. This was an unprovoked attack and the police caught the man who has since been released. He attended the accident and emergency department and the bite was cleaned and dressed. It was superficial and did not require sutures. He was put on antibiotics and given a tetanus toxoid booster. He knows nothing about his attacker, but is very worried about the risk of AIDS. He requests an HIV test. What do you advise at this time?

In cases of violence and assault, information which may help to assess risk of blood borne disease includes:

• knowledge of past medical history of assailant or contact

• whether others involved consent to tests for HIV or hepatitis B

• social history which puts contact/assailant at high risk of HIV or hepatitis B infection

[665]

This patient is distressed and frightened. Would you counsel him and do the test if he decided to have it? What is the risk of HIV infection in this case? (665)

Why should this patient be the one to have any tests? The police know who his attacker was. The assailant should be asked to provide relevant medical and social information. He could also be asked if he was willing to have blood tests to clarify the risk of infection.

Violence may cause wounds that are contaminated with someone else's blood and the protocol for a needle stick injury may be appropriate as there is a risk of blood borne disease [666]

If violence or assault has resulted in a risk of HIV infection, counselling should mention the option of taking blood at four monthly intervals for storage and subsequent testing if required [667]

If violence or assault has resulted in a risk of HIV or hepatitis B infection:

- an accelerated course of hepatitis B immunisation should be given

- blood should be taken for storage for HIV status if needed later

- a further blood test should be done in six months time to check anti-HBs levels [668]

It is important to obtain detailed information about the attack. The patient remembers that the man had some blood on his lip before he bit him. This increases the risk of infection (666). The decision to have an HIV test is never urgent, and there is always time to reconsider provided the options in rule 667 are considered.

Decisions about HIV testing could be postponed until he has got over the shock. He can then be counselled about the issues involved. It also gives time for his solicitor to obtain information from his assailant. Blood should, however, be taken for storage to establish his HIV status at the time of the attack.

What other disease might be contracted as a result of this assault? There is also a risk of hepatitis B infection. What can be done to try and prevent this disease? (668)

The patient initially saw the trainee who asked her trainer for advice. If expert advice is needed who should be asked? Options include the Communicable Disease Surveillance Centre, a pathologist, or infectious disease specialist. The opinion of the pathologist at a hospital that dealt with a lot of HIV and hepatitis infection was to take blood for storage and subsequent HIV testing if needed, and for the patient to have an accelerated course of hepatitis B immunisation. There should be a follow up blood test at six months to check anti-HBs levels.

Case 47

A woman who is 37 weeks' pregnant comes to the antenatal clinic saying that for the last two days she has not felt any movements. This is her first pregnancy. She has attended all her antenatal clinic appointments and there were no high risk factors; everything has been normal throughout the pregnancy. She feels well. On examination the fetal heart beat cannot be heard, and she admitted to much reduced movement for a few days and not feeling any movement for the last 24 hours. She was admitted to hospital. A stillbirth was diagnosed and she delivered a macerated but otherwise normal fetus. A hospital discharge note is received saying she was discharged two days ago. What is your management?

In cases of unexpected death or stillbirth, a home visit should be done to provide bereavement counselling, support, and to re-establish confidence   [105]

In cases of unexpected death or stillbirth, recent patient management should be reviewed to identify preventable factors   [563]

Some antenatal complications and stillbirths can be prevented if women know what to do when problems such as reduced movements, bleeding, oedema, or severe headaches develop during pregnancy   [733]

Others who need to be informed about deaths and stillbirths may include doctors, nurses, health visitors, midwives, appointment and transport staff, and records should indicate who has been told   [630]

Should a home visit be done and, if so, what would be its objectives? (105)

Before seeing the patient, it might be advisable to obtain the answers to questions that could be anticipated (563).

Perhaps there were no obvious risk factors, but what about her own response to reduced fetal movements? Was this appropriate or not? (733)

This is not the time to ask why she did not seek help earlier. Did the shared care antenatal book contain advice about what to do if she noticed reduced or absent movements? She needs bereavement counselling and help to deal with her guilt about not seeking help earlier. Management at this time includes communication with others involved in the care of this patient (630).

Hospital staff do not always inform all the relevant people. It is the GP's responsibility to ensure that this happens. It is important to give this patient a follow up appointment.

Case 48

A woman aged 52 comes to see you because of persistent pain in her right hip following a slight fall three weeks before. She has no past history of serious illness and has full movement of the hip. There are no abnormal signs apart from the limp on walking; otherwise she feels well. A radiograph of the hip showed a subcapsular undisplaced fracture. The orthopaedic registrar felt surgery was not indicated as it seemed to be healing. A follow up orthopaedic appointment has been given. What is your management?

This patient has fractured her hip at the age of 52. This was surprising in view of the minimal trauma involved. Is she more vulnerable to fractures than other women of the

---

Management decisions must be related to one or more of the following objectives:

- prevention of illness
- prevention of disability in curable illness
- prevention of further disability in chronic diseases
- prevention of recurrence or relapse
- prevention of death [64]

Osteoporosis is a preventable disease and women at risk include those with a history of:

- early menopause before the age of 45
- oophorectomy before the age of 45
- family history of osteoporosis
- previous fractures
- use of oral steroids [764]

Long term medication may be necessary to prevent recurrence or relapse of certain diseases [712]

Women need information about the effects that antibiotics, diarrhoea, or vomiting have on the Pill, and the need for additional methods of birth control at such times [765]

same age? What "at risk" group might she belong to? Could this fracture have been prevented? (64)

What observations might suggest an increased risk of fracture in a woman of this age? Is there a risk of osteoporosis? Is she hormonally challenged or can the word menopause still be used? (764)

How could osteoporosis be prevented in high risk groups of women? (712)

In the absence of any contraindication, women such as this patient should be given hormone replacement therapy. The goal for this patient is to prevent further fractures. How could the diagnosis of osteoporosis be confirmed? A normal radiograph does not exclude this diagnosis. She was referred to the department of nuclear medicine where a bone density examination showed evidence of osteoporosis. She was put on long term hormone replacement therapy.

Case 49

A woman aged 25 consults because she has developed diarrhoea and vomiting for the last 36 hours. She now says the vomiting has stopped and the diarrhoea is less than it was. There is no abdominal pain or blood in the stools. She has no past history of serious illness and asks for a certificate for another couple of days, after which she thinks she will feel able to return to work. What is your management?

It can be difficult to remember that prevention is relevant to every consultation. Here the failure to educate this patient about the effects of her illness on the effectiveness of birth control could result in an unwanted pregnancy (765).

Case 50

A man aged 26 comes for a certificate to return to work. He was injured in a road traffic accident. He had a fractured tibia and fibula and a ruptured spleen which was removed. He has made a good recovery and is now fit to return to his job as a manager in the local supermarket. What is your management at this time?

The goals of this consultation include providing a certificate as requested, but will the doctor recognise the risks that splenectomy presents to this patient? (896)

Did the hospital staff explain about the risk of infection and was he given written instructions on how to prevent such complications? Who is responsible for ensuring that preventive measures are undertaken? The surgical directorate should have a policy and written information needs to be given to such patients. What is the role of the GP?

> Patients who have had a splenectomy must be:
>
> - counselled about the risk of infection and its prevention
> - immunised against pneumococcal, *Haemophilus influenzae*, and meningococcal infections
> - provided with long term antibiotic prophylaxis (amoxycillin)
> - given an information card to help identify early signs of sepsis and take appropriate action
> - given amoxycillin for self treatment of early signs of infection [896]
>
> *BMJ* 1994;**308**:131–3

In a recent review of 557 patients only 87 had been immunised against pneumococcal infection. Of 55 who died, six died of pneumococcal sepsis and none had received any prophylaxis.[2] In fact, few received any prophylaxis or advice. The options are those shown in the box.

There is clear evidence that prophylactic measures decrease the risk of severe infection in this group of patients. GPs should keep a register of patients who have had a splenectomy. A decision needs to be made about the need for a practice policy for prevention of serious infections in such patients.[3]

> - National campaign
> - Surgical policy in hospitals
> - GP education
> - Register of such patients in hospitals and general practices

Case 51

Your practice is fund holding and you wish to finalise your contracts for surgical treatment with local providers. The day surgery and inpatient requirements have been identified, and issues relating to postoperative prescribing and communication have been clarified. Quality criteria need to be incorporated into the contract. What factors could be considered at this stage?

The answer to this question will depend on the objectives for care before, during, and after surgery. One of the most important goals is to prevent complications (191).

> All other things being equal, select the surgeon who takes active measures to reduce risk of pulmonary emboli [191]

Low dose heparin and aspirin have been shown to reduce the incidence of this serious complication for certain groups of patients.[4-6] Quality criteria should include the use of antiplatelet measures to reduce the risk of thrombosis and pulmonary emboli after surgery.

Prevention of osteomalacia

Osteomalacia is a completely preventable disease. The high risk patients are pregnant Asian women. Treatment with calcium and vitamin D tablets should be routine practice in all antenatal clinics where these high risk groups of patients are seen. It should also be part of antenatal community care for women who are seen at home by midwives, but who may be unwilling to attend the hospital clinics. Why do so few hospitals have a policy to prevent this disease and ensure that it is carried out in practice? This question should be raised by the GP representative on the obstetric and gynaecology clinical directorate. Prevention of osteomalacia should be built into the provider contracts by purchasers on behalf of their Asian patients in the community.

Stopping smoking

Initial advice from practice nurses to stop smoking is of doubtful effectiveness, but systematic follow up of motivated patients by nurses can achieve a significant three month sustained rate of smoking cessation.[7] Analysis of results of 28 randomised trials of nicotine replacement therapy has shown that this enables 15% of smokers who seek help to stop smoking.[8] This evidence should affect the management decisions of nurses and doctors when confronted with motivated patients who wish to stop smoking.

Prevention of maternal mortality

Of the 238 maternal deaths during 1988–90 15–17% were caused by pulmonary embolism. Anticoagulant prophylaxis at caesarean section has been shown to prevent maternal mortality from pulmonary embolism, yet this is not routine practice in most obstetric units.[9] GPs must ensure that preventive measures are built into the contracts of purchasers of obstetric services.

107

Conclusion

Prevention is still a frequently overlooked goal. Only when it has become as important to our thinking as making a diagnosis will this objective really become part of every patient consultation.

1 Stott N, Davis R. The exceptional potential in every primary care consultation. *Journal of the Royal College of General Practitioners* 1979; **29**:201–5.
2 McMullin M, Johnston G. Long term management of patients after splenectomy. *BMJ* 1993;**307**:1372–3.
3 Kinnersley P, Wilkinson G, Srinivasan J. Pneumococcal vaccination after splenectomy: survey of hospital and primary care records. *BMJ* 1993;**307**:1398–9.
4 Thromboembolic Risk Factors (THRIFT) Consensus Group. Risk of prophylaxis for venous thromboembolism in hospital patients. *BMJ* 1992;**305**:567–74.
5 Antiplatelet Trialists' Collaboration. Collaborative overview of randomised trials of antiplatelet treatment. III. Reduction in venous thrombosis and pulmonary embolism by antiplatelet prophylaxis among surgical and medical patients. *BMJ* 1994;**308**:235–46.
6 Underwood M, More R. The aspirin papers. *BMJ* 1994;**308**:71–2.
7 ICRF general practice research group. The effectiveness of transdermal nicotine patch in helping heavy smokers to stop smoking: results of a randomised trial in UK general practice. *BMJ* 1993;**306**:1304–8.
8 Tang LJ, Law M, Wald N. How effective is nicotine replacement therapy in helping people to stop smoking? *BMJ* 1994;**308**:21–6.
9 Department of Health. *Report on confidential enquiries into maternal deaths in the United Kingdom 1988–1990*. London: HMSO, 1994.

III Special problems

15 Decisions about children

The Children Act has profound implications for decisions that GPs make about the management of children's problems. The best way to understand how the Act operates is to consider first what it was designed to do.

Contents of the Act

The Children Act relates to the issues in the box. These are described in detail in the Department of Health guidelines.[1]

- Public and private law
- Parental responsibility and parents' rights
- Providing services
- Protecting children
- Looking after children away from home

Implications for the health service

There is a duty on health authorities and NHS Trusts to cooperate with social service departments. Interagency cooperation is needed both to protect children and to provide them with the services they need. The guiding principle is one of partnership with parents based on agreement. Greater collaboration is required among social service departments, health professionals, parents, other carers, and children, in meeting the needs of children in the care of social services and other agencies. The rules in this book have been derived after careful study of the Act together with a social worker who has special experience in this field.

This chapter lists problems that have presented to GPs. Most of the rules for these cases have been derived from the Children Act. Each case lists a few relevant rules but others may be equally applicable. Try to make your own management decisions before reading the rules.

Case 52

A foster mother brings a girl aged 14 to evening surgery. The foster mother says she has been accommodated by the local authority in a foster home for the last three months. She is worried because she is sexually active. The girl confirms this. Both are requesting that she be put on the contraceptive pill. What is your management?

Consent to treat a child in social services care involves identifying the wishes and feelings of:

- the child

- the parents

- anyone else who has parental responsibility

- others whose wishes and feeling the authority considers to be relevant

and it is the social worker's responsibility to obtain consent from those with parental responsibility [813]

When a child is the subject of a care order, parental responsibility is shared between the social services and the parents themselves, and the Department of Social Services has the power to decide how much the parents may exercise their parental responsibilities [814]

Case 53

A boy aged 12 years comes to morning surgery requesting holiday injections for a school holiday abroad in two weeks time. You ask if he has an adult with him to consent for these injections. He says that his mother's partner is outside and he will agree. What is your management?

Consent for treatment of child is a parental responsibility and if:

- married at time of child's birth, they shall each have parental responsibility

- not married at time of child's birth, the mother shall have parental responsibility

- the father shall not have parental responsibility unless he acquires it in accordance with the provisions of the Children Act 1989

- where more than one person has parental responsibility each may act alone [826]

Case 54

A young girl aged 14 comes to request the Pill. She is having unprotected sex and wants to ensure that she does not become pregnant. She says that it is impossible to discuss this with her parents as they would be very angry with her boyfriend who is aged 19. She seems competent and sensible. What is your management?

A doctor can give contraceptive advice or treatment without parental knowledge or consent to a child under 16, provided:

- she has sufficient intelligence to understand what is proposed
- she has been counselled on the advisability of involving her parents or a person in *loco parentis*
- contraception is considered to be in the patient's best interest [797]

If a competent patient refuses consent to communicate with a relative or other third party, the doctor must respect the patient's wishes for confidentiality, and this is particularly relevant where the patient is a child under 16 [782]

If a competent child gives consent to treatment, provision of that treatment is lawful whether the parent gives consent or refuses, but the doctor is not obliged to treat. [795]

Case 55

You are looking after a child aged eight who has developed idiopathic thrombocytopenic purpura. She needs a blood transfusion. Her parents disagree about the need for this treatment. Her mother wants to do what the doctors think is best, but the father is against a blood transfusion. The consultant telephones you to discuss this issue and see if you can persuade the father to change his mind. What is your advice?

Consent for treatment of child is a parental responsibility and if:

- married at time of child's birth, they shall each have parental responsibility
- not married at time of child's birth, the mother shall have parental responsibility
- the father shall not have parental responsibility unless he acquires it in accordance with the provisions of the Children Act 1989
- where more than one person has parental responsibility each may act alone [826]

If parents disagree with each other about treatment, the doctor only requires the consent of one authorised person, competent child, or parent for treatment to be legally provided [794]

If a child who is too immature to consent needs a life saving or emergency treatment, and the parents refuse consent, or no other valid consent can be obtained, doctors can treat the child but should obtain:

- written supporting opinion of a medical colleague that life would be endangered if treatment is withheld
- acknowledgement from the parents, preferably in writing or before a witness, that the danger had been explained to them and that their consent was still withheld [796]

Case 56

A mother aged 30 comes to evening surgery. After some hesitation she says that she is afraid that her husband is planning to take her young daughter, aged seven years, out of the country to have her circumcised according to his cultural tradition. She does not know what to do, and asks your advice.

The Prohibition of Female Circumcision Act 1989 makes this procedure an offence except on specific physical or mental health grounds, and if there is a risk that this may happen, the social services has a duty to investigate what action, if any, should be taken to safeguard the child's welfare [815]

If a girl is thought to have been or is at risk of circumcision a Child Protection Investigation should take place involving social services and the Police Child Protection Team, and such children may be placed on the Child Protection Register [816]

A girl who has been circumcised might not be placed on the Child Protection Register, but should be offered counselling and medical help, and steps need to be taken to prevent similar harm to other children in the family [817]

Significant harm is described in the Children Act which defines harm, development, health, and ill treatment (see section 31) [829]

The objectives of a child protection referral to social services are:

- to clarify the facts about referral

- to identify areas of concern

- to assess whether there are grounds for concern

- to identify any risk factors

- to discover any reasonable cause to suspect that a child is suffering or at risk of significant harm, abuse, or neglect

- to decide if it is safe to leave the child in the household [883]

Anxieties expressed by parents about the association between intervention by the Department of Social Services and the diagnosis of potential child abuse will necessitate open and honest discussion between parents, carers, Department of Social Services, and health service staff about the role of the individual agencies and their agreed procedures for transfer of information [889]

Case 57

You are contacted by a social worker who has just begun to work with James, a boy aged nine years with growth failure and renal disease, who is partially sighted. The family live in overcrowded housing and the social worker's task involves trying to assess James's special needs and also to help the family reduce the frequent failed medical appointments for dental, optical checks, ENT, and speech and language therapy. The social worker tells you that she is also very concerned about the youngest sibling Sarah, aged seven, who is starting fires and becoming hard to control. She feels that this is a family that may need child guidance referral and wonders what you think. On reviewing the records James has been seen by many different doctors in the practice, and Sarah has only attended once. What is your management?

A child in need is someone who, without provision of social services:

- is unlikely to achieve or maintain, or have opportunity to achieve or maintain, a reasonable standard of health or development
- is likely to have significantly impaired health or development or
- is disabled   [885]

Children with disabilities or special needs may benefit from an interagency plan to ensure that needs are met and duplication avoided; this should specify:

- measurable goals
- resources and services to be provided
- allocation of responsibilities
- arrangements for monitoring and review   [820]

Children with disabilities require coordinated support from a wide range of services and continual reassessment of needs and response to treatment, and the responsibilities of the GP, health visitor, social worker, etc, need to be clearly defined   [818]

Children with disabilities may have special housing needs and the Children Act provides for the cooperation of housing authorities, social services departments, local educational authorities, district health authorities, and NHS trusts   [819]

The Children Act states that if a child is suspected to be at risk of violence, abuse, or "significant harm," the social services has a duty to investigate and decide whether any action needs to be taken to safeguard the child's welfare   [822]

Every local authority shall open and maintain a register of disabled children within their area   [821]

Significant harm is described in the Children Act which defines harm, development, health, and ill treatment (see section 31)   [829]

Case 58

Parents who both have learning difficulties come to surgery with their children aged 14, 12, nine, and seven years. The family are loving and close, but the children are very dirty and smelly. They are obese, their hair is matted, and the skin looks as if they have scabies. The mother has brought them because they have lice. The parents also say that they have difficulties coping with money and that the children have problems coping with school. What is your management?

Children with disabilities or special needs may benefit from an interagency plan to ensure that needs are met and duplication avoided, this should specify:

- measurable goals
- resources and services to be provided
- allocation of responsibilities
- arrangements for monitoring and review   [820]

The social services are responsible for safeguarding and promoting the welfare of children in need within their families by providing a level of services appropriate to those needs   [884]

A child in need is someone who, without provision of social services:

- is unlikely to achieve or maintain, or have opportunity to achieve or maintain, a reasonable standard of health or development
- is likely to have significantly impaired health or development or
- is disabled   [885]

Case 59

A woman aged 58 complains that she has become very depressed. She feels that life holds no future for her. She says that, since the divorce of her son and his wife, she can no longer see her grandchildren. Previously they were in daily contact. She has tried to arrange visits but these have been unsuccessful. She feels that she cannot go on without seeing them. She asks for some treatment that might "put more life in me." What is your management?

The right of access to children may be acquired via a court "contact order" which requires the person with whom a child lives, or is to live, to allow the child to visit or stay with the person named in the order, or for that person and the child to have contact with each other   [825]

A grandparent may seek, under the Children Act, the right to maintain contact with grandchildren and may benefit from legal advice if such access is denied   [824]

Case 60

A man comes to see you because he is concerned about his relationship with the woman he has been living with for the last five years. They are not married but have twins aged 18 months. They are talking about separating although they have not made a final decision about this, and are receiving some help from Relate. He is very worried that, if they do separate, he will not be allowed access to his children. He has been told that, although he is the father, he does not have parental right of access because they are not married. "What can I do, doctor?"

> Natural fathers may acquire parental responsibility by written agreement with the mother in a format laid down in a statutory instrument (No. 1478 of 1991) signed by both parties, then registered at Somerset House [898]

> Natural fathers may also seek a court order for parental responsibility if the mother does not agree, but the court also has the power to remove it later on [899]

Case 61

A woman aged 42 has twice left her home for a woman's refuge following domestic violence from her husband. She brings her son aged seven years to surgery. He has a large bruise on his thigh. She says this was caused by a fall in the park. She wants to know if any special treatment is needed. She seems frightened and has an emerging bruise on her upper cheek which she says she got walking into a door. The child is silent but than talks about falling against his bed at home.

> Whenever non-accidental injury is suspected, the child's welfare is top priority and the GP has a duty to involve the social services [827]

> The necessity for referral to social services may be difficult for some families to accept and the GP may be the most appropriate person to:
> - identify unresolved anger and
> - explain why such a referral must be made [835]

Case 62

The trainee has been telephoned by the duty social worker to say that a child aged two years, who is a patient, has been found alone in the family flat. The child was found soaked in urine, undernourished, and with considerable bruising to the face and body. The parents' whereabouts are unknown. He says that the family were unknown to them and there appear to be no other relatives. They are seeking an Emergency Protection order today. He asks if you can help with any background or medical information. She felt that this was confidential information, but asks for your opinion. What is your response?

> The GP has a statutory duty to provide confidential information to social services, educational, housing, and health authorities, who must cooperate with each other in supporting children and their families [828]

117

Case 63

You are consulted by a girl aged 15. She has a green vaginal discharge and the swab you took grew *Trichomonas* sp. She is sexually active and you explain the need for birth control and the use of condoms to prevent infections. You encourage her to discuss the need for treatment with her parents but she says that this is impossible to do. You treat her infection and also give her enough medication for her partner. She understands the need for both to be treated. She is on the contraceptive pill which she has obtained from the family planning clinic. A week later, her mother comes to see you. She has found an empty bottle of antibiotics and wants to know why her daughter consulted and what is wrong. You explain that this is confidential but she requests access to her daughter's records. What is your response?

Parents may have access to a child's record if the child is able and willing to give consent or if the child is unable to understand the nature of the application, but access is considered in the child's best interests, and information that the child thought would be kept confidential should not be revealed [809]

The Children Act 1989 states that the social services may provide accommodation for any child in need within their area (even though a person who has parental responsibility is able to provide accommodation) if failure to do so could seriously endanger the child's welfare [830]

Case 64

A mother comes to talk about her son aged 16. She is very angry because he has been destroying the home and stealing. She says that he drinks, does not come home often at night, and is sleeping rough. She suspects that he goes up to the West End of London and has a very strange group of friends. She says "I am at the end of my tether." She says that he will have to go as his drinking and behaviour tantrums are a danger to his step brother and sister aged five and three years, and that all this is "doing my head in." She says that her son and stepfather do not get on, and this makes it worse. She wanted him to come to the surgery but he refused. "What can I do, doctor?" What is your management?

> The Children Act 1989 states that the social services may provide accommodation for any child in need within their area (even though a person who has parental responsibility is able to provide accommodation) if failure to do so could seriously endanger the child's welfare
>
> [830]

> The social services are responsible for safeguarding and promoting the welfare of children in need within their families by providing a level of services appropriate to those needs   [884]

Case 65

The health visitor attached to your practice comes to you because she has just visited a young mother and learned that she is also caring for a neighbour's two children while the neighbour works. The young mother says she likes being a child minder although she does not get paid much. All the children seem well cared for. The health visitor asks if she should do anything about this?

> A person caring for a child acts as a child minder if:
>
> - they look after one or more children under the age of eight years for reward
> - the period spent looking after children in any day exceeds two hours
>
> The social services have a statutory duty to inspect and keep a register of all child minders   [877]

Case 66

A person who:
- is the parent
- a relative
- has parental responsibility or
- is a foster parent

does not act as a child minder when caring for a child   [878]

An elderly grandparent brings her granddaughter to surgery for her three year developmental check. She confides that she is very worried. She cares daily for her granddaughter while her parents work. Her neighbour has told her that she could be acting as an unregistered childminder and she does not know what to do. She says that her daughter has a large debt and cannot stop working. She asks your advice about what she ought to do. What is your management?

Case 67

If a mother has a serious mental illness, which appears to impair her child care, the GP must refer to social services who will assess the risk, and offer help and support following a multiagency meeting   [831]

A single mother aged 22 who is a known schizophrenic comes to surgery with her son aged two years who has a rash and asthma. She seems vague and indicates that her neighbours are causing many problems and want to take her son away from her. She has had three previous admissions, one voluntary and two under section. You treat the child's eczema and ask her how she is. She admits to having stopped her injections three months previously but says "I am not mad if that's what you think." The health visitor who is at the surgery confirms that mother and son live alone and do not have family support. What is your management?

Case 68

A health visitor attached to your practice comes for advice. She has just visited the upstairs neighbour of a family registered with you. Three years ago the two older daughters in this family were found to have suffered sexual abuse by their stepfather. He left the home, was prosecuted, and given a prison sentence. The neighbour has told the health visitor that she has seen the stepfather leaving the flat in the early mornings. What is your management?

When a doctor suspects a child is being physically or sexually abused, the duty to disclose information to a third party (social worker or police) takes priority over the right to confidentiality   [569]

If the GP suspects that a child is at risk of sexual abuse, the social worker must be urgently contacted as the social services have a duty to investigate and decide whether further action should be taken   [832]

Case 69

A mother comes to surgery with her oldest son aged 13 who has Down's syndrome, and a mental age of six. He has limited vision. She explains that he is home for the summer from residential school but she has become very concerned about his recent behaviour, and talks of "secrets" when being supervised in the bath. After much embarrassment she explains he has been masturbating in front of the family and has asked other children to "lick his penis" and "fuck." She says that this is all very new behaviour and she does not know how to handle it. What is your management?

> If children with learning difficulties present with behaviour problems, which could be either emerging sexuality or sexual abuse, the social services have a duty to investigate and such cases should be referred to the Department of Social Services   [834]

Case 70

The school nurse of the local primary school telephones to say that she is concerned about a boy aged seven years who is your patient. The child seems to be losing weight, seems miserable, and is very irritable in school. She has tried to contact the parents to arrange a school medical but gets no response. She has approached the teachers and social services who have both tried to contact the parents. The family are refusing to speak to them because of anger over a referral and investigation of a bruise sustained by an older child which was later found to be caused accidentally. You see from the notes that the child has not been seen for two years. You invite the parents to the surgery but there is no response. You do a home visit, but the mother comes to the door and refuses to let you in. What is your management?

> When children are suspected to be at risk of neglect or abuse their welfare is paramount and the social services have a duty to investigate; a Child Protection Conference may recommend an application to the court for a Child Assessment Order   [836]

Case 71

A mother comes to evening surgery with her two daughters aged 12 and seven years. She says the younger daughter has been very quiet and tearful lately, and has now told her older sister that an older boy in the local playground has been "touching her minnie" and has been asking her to touch him. The mother is distraught and tells you that her husband would know how to deal with it but he is abroad at the moment. She says she does not know what to do. What is your management?

> Children who are suspected of sexually abusing other children may themselves have been abused, and the appropriate child protection procedures should be followed in respect of both the victim and the abuser   [886]

> Where child abuse is alleged to have been done by another child or young person, the appropriate child protection procedures should be followed   [879]

Case 72

> Urgent discussions with the Department of Social Services or an interagency meeting may be needed to assess the risk to the unborn child; if there is sufficient concern a pre-birth child protection case conference may be considered   [880]

A woman five months' pregnant who has just moved into the area consults you for the first time. She says that this is her third pregnancy and, although the other two children were adopted, this one is going to be different. You organise her blood tests and antenatal booking clinic appointment. After she has left the surgery, you learn from your practice partner that he remembers that her other two children had to be taken into care and later adopted following severe emotional abuse and neglect. What is your management?

Case 73

A woman aged 23 is the last patient in an evening surgery and is seen with her children aged 13 months and five years. She has been living in a hostel for battered women. The baby has a cough but is not febrile or wheezy. A child in the hostel has recently had whooping cough. She has not had her children immunised. You notice a superficial first degree burn on the baby's leg which mother says was the result of an accidental scald three days previously. There are also a few old bruises on the upper arms which were caused by "a fall." She has never seen a social worker or health visitor since being in the hostel. Tomorrow she moves out to new accommodation 9 miles away. What is your management?

In the assessment of risk of non-accidental injury the following observations are relevant:

- account inconsistent with injuries
- delay in seeking help
- risk factors, for example, single isolated young parent
- past history of burns, fractures, child abuse in family, a child on child protection register at any time
- bruises at different stages, finger/thumb marks, circular burns, torn frenulum [360]

In cases of suspected child abuse or neglect, useful information includes past family history, whether any child had been placed on the child protection register in this or any other district, the previous GP's knowledge of family if the patient is new to the practice; discussions with social services must also be undertaken [81]

The current GP, in conjunction with the Department of Social Services, have a responsibility to organise follow up of high risk, suspected non-accidental injury, or child abuse cases who move to a new area [256]

Case 74

A mother brings her daughter aged six years who has a vaginal discharge. A swab is sent and mother returns with the child four days later. The swab grew gonococci. There is no past history of serious illness or psychological problems, and there is no record of any child of this family being on the child protection register. What is your management?

After an allegation or disclosure of actual or suspected child sexual abuse the management responsibilities of the GP include:

- keeping detailed records
- avoiding leading questions that might contaminate evidence
- minimising need to re-interview child
- urgent discussion with staff of local social services to decide if an expert interview and examination is needed, and, if so, which relative should accompany child
- discussing with parents their worries and anxieties and informing them of what is going to happen
- sharing follow up management decisions with social services [576]

Whenever non-accidental injury is suspected, the child's welfare is top priority and the GP has a duty to involve the social services [827]

In cases of suspected child abuse, sexual abuse, or non-accidental injury, management should follow the policy of the local area child protection committee (ACPC) and guidelines, as outlined by the district health authority or the Department of Health [449]

The procedures of other agencies need to be understood to ensure that a full investigatory process for suspected child abuse or non-accidental injury is not initiated prematurely [571]

When referring to social services it is essential to have a coordinated approach and avoid unplanned contact with child's parents or carers which might put the child at risk of threat or pressure to retract or to conceal abuse [882]

Sexual abuse in children is usually followed by guilt, anxiety, and fear of permanent damage; after identification of the problem, follow up support is needed to resolve these sequelae [450]

The objectives of a child protection referral to social services are:

- to clarify the facts about referral
- to identify areas of concern
- to assess whether there are grounds for concern
- to identify any risk factors
- to discover any reasonable cause to suspect that a child is suffering or at risk of significant harm, abuse, or neglect
- to decide if it is safe to leave the child in the household [883]

Case 75

A mother brings daughter aged 10 with a sore throat, and vaginal discomfort and discharge. She says the throat has been sore for two days and there is a yellow vaginal discharge. It is 6.30 p.m. on Friday. There is pus on both tonsils and enlarged cervical glands. There is no past history of serious illness or medical or social problems. What is your management?

> Risk of child sexual abuse or non-accidental injury is likely to be increased if:
> - parent was abused or
> - sib was abused or
> - sib was on child protection register [568]

> In cases of suspected child abuse or neglect, useful information includes past family history, whether any child had been placed on the child protection register in this or any other district, the previous GP's knowledge of family if the patient is new to practice; discussions with social services must also be undertaken [481]

> In a child with a yellow vaginal discharge:
> - take a full history
> - identify risk factors in the patient and family which might indicate child sexual abuse
> - do a full examination and
> - send swabs to exclude gonococcal infection [731]

> There should be a practice policy to indicate, on all family members' problem lists, if any child was ever put on the child protection register [362]

> Children aged 12 and over cannot be adopted without their consent, and children who are mature enough will take part in their own adoption proceedings, with legal representation [894]

Case 76

A child aged 12 is brought by foster parents who say that the social services have arranged for his adoption by a couple who the child has met twice but does not like very much. He would like to be adopted by his foster parents with whom he has been living for the last two years. They want to adopt him but the Department of Social Services say that they are not suitable as they are white and he is Afro-Caribbean. The foster parents feel that he has become depressed and anxious and want you to support his desire to be adopted by them. What is your management?

> Children aged 12 and over cannot be adopted without their consent, and children who are mature enough will take part in their own adoption proceedings, with legal representation [894]

> In assessing parental suitability for adoption, the most important factor is the judgement made about their ability to help and support the child, and although ethnicity and culture need to be considered they are not decisive (new Adoption Bill 1994–95 session of parliament) [895]

A full analysis of these cases, as in other chapters, is available in a special teaching format from me on request. It forms a comprehensive introduction to suspected child abuse and discusses the application of rules derived from the Children Act to a wide range of problems seen in general practice.

1 Department of Health. *Working together – under the Children Act 1989*, London, HMSO, 1991.
2 Childcare Co-ordinators Unit. *Child protection precedures*, Lewisham Social Services, 1993. (Excellent guidelines.)

16 HIV/AIDS

Patients with HIV/AIDS present special ethical, legal, medical, psychological, and social problems, involving patients, partners, carers, and health staff. GPs share the care of these vulnerable patients who often present difficult management dilemmas.

Case 77

A man aged 30 comes with a cough and cold. He has been gay for many years but now plans to get married. He has no anxieties about this but you wonder whether it would be sensible to raise the question of HIV risks. What is your management?

Premarital counselling is important for some patients with chronic diseases or disabilities, or who are at risk of genetic or infective diseases [634]

He may have already considered the risks and had an HIV test done. Alternatively he may have considered this but felt too embarrassed to ask for advice. The need for premarital counselling is becoming more widely recognised (634).

A partner or contact has a right to know about risk of exposure to an infectious disease [606]

There is another person to consider and she also has rights (606). If this right is denied, the patient should be aware of the possible outcomes (344).

A patient who decides not to inform others about the risk of infection must recognise that this decision may have serious outcomes for partner and future children [344]

This patient had been unable to confront this issue. After counselling he decided to have an HIV test. This was negative and there had been no homosexual activity for the last 18 months. He was grateful that the subject had been discussed.

Case 78

A woman aged 27 comes for advice. She has had a bisexual boyfriend for four years. This relationship has now ended. She wonders whether she ought to have an HIV test because she does not want to be a risk to any new boy-friend she may have in the future. "What do you think, doctor?"

Patients need information on the medical, social, psychological, occupational, insurance, and mortgage implications of a positive HIV test before deciding whether to give informed consent for it to be done   [395]

Informed consent is needed before doing an HIV test. The patient needs to understand the implications of having this investigation (395). She needs to understand the significance of a negative test result (397).

To know if recent exposure to sexually transmitted disease has caused infection, two negative test results are needed three months apart, with no risk of infection during this period
[397]

Would she be able to cope with a positive result? This is a very important question and a review of past mental illness would be relevant (490).

The relative risk of suicide in an AIDS patient is very high (over 66 times greater than that of the general population) and its occurrence is most probable early in the course of the illness
JAMA 1988;**259**:1333–7   [490]

Another implication of HIV testing relates to insurance (597). There are HIV/AIDS counsellors in most districts, and all genitourinary clinics provide counselling. This patient could be referred to a specialist counsellor or the GP may have the skills needed to undertake this task. If the HIV test is done at a genitourinary clinic, the results will not be sent to the GP and the notes will not record that the test was done (525).

When counselling for HIV tests, a checklist of points should include the fact that, if records indicate a test was done, even if the result was negative, insurance may be refused   [597]

It may take more than one consultation to counsel a patient about an HIV test, and the patient may want to discuss its implications with others before making an informed decision in a calm state of mind   [525]

To prevent hepatitis, the GP should use Department of Health guidelines to identify high risk behaviours, occupations, and groups who need to be screened and possibly immunised [529]

High risk of HIV infection is accompanied by high risk of being a hepatitis B carrier and, if informed consent is given for an HIV test, the patient usually agrees to a hepatitis B test as well [528]

What other investigations might also be indicated? (529) Her partner's lifestyle increases the risk of other infectious diseases (528). The patient should be told why a hepatitis test would be useful. If it were positive, any new partner could be offered hepatitis B immunisation. Her liver function tests should be done and, if abnormal, she should be referred for possible interferon treatment. Counselling must include advice about reducing the risk of HIV infection. Behaviour modification and advice about safe sex are essential to prevent the spread of this infection.

Case 79

A report from the accident and emergency department states that one of your patients attended with severe lacerations following a road traffic accident. He required many sutures. You know that he is HIV positive but there is no mention of this in the report. Do you take any further action?

It may be important to clarify what guidelines are provided to accident and emergency staff and medical students to reduce occupational risks of hepatitis and HIV infection, and whether or not they are observed [516]

Informed consent to disclose confidential information may be given if the patient understands the importance of information for the safety of others who may be at risk, including doctors and nurses [515]

It is possible that he did not mention his HIV status to the hospital staff. In a perfect world doctors would suture everyone as if they were HIV positive. In practice this does not always happen. If it was not mentioned, he needs to recognise why doctors need this information. The patient was asked to make an appointment. He did not mention his HIV status and said he was sutured by a medical student who did not wear gloves. He had felt too embarrassed to tell staff about his HIV status, but agreed that it was in their interest to know. It seemed reasonable to discuss the risks taken by the student, with the accident and emergency consultant (516).

The consultant said that students were given instructions to always wear gloves when doing suturing, but they did not always do so. She was told about the student who did not wear gloves for an HIV positive patient. The consultant asked for the patient's name so that his HIV status could be recorded in the notes. Is this an acceptable request? If the name is given, what grounds are there for breaching confidentiality? (515)

The patient gave consent for the consultant to be informed of his HIV status. The student needs further instruction about the importance of taking infectious disease control measures. He also has the right to know of his possible exposure to HIV infection. Management could follow the protocol for a needle stick injury. Someone must be responsible for the follow up and counselling of this student. It could be the accident and emergency consultant, the student's GP, or the consultant responsible for student health. His hepatitis B immunisation status should also be checked.

Case 80

A man aged 25 lives alone, weighs 20 stone, is HIV positive and has epilepsy. He has recently had three fits which were followed by a short period of uncontrolled aggression before a post ictal period of unconsciousness. During the last two fits he fell and cut himself, and a neighbour came in to help him and to dress the cuts. He is complying with his medication and has come for a repeat prescription. What is your management?

A differential diagnosis must be made of treatment failure which includes factors related to diagnosis, natural history, presence of complications, patient's behaviour, information given, treatment, dosage, compliance, prevention of recurrence, coexisting diseases and their treatment, and follow up provided [591]

A recall system is needed for safe follow up of patients who:

- are on long term medication
- need periodic investigations or examinations
- are on an at risk register [194]

The three important management objectives are to reduce the frequency of fits, ensure prompt treatment when they occur, and prevent spread of infection to others. In this case, treatment is not controlling the disease (591, 194).

Patients with a repeat prescription card for long term medication need regular follow up to assess whether

- management is still effective
- treatment is still being taken
- indications for treatment have changed
- all the drugs are still needed
- dosages are appropriate
- side effects have occurred
- drug interactions are likely
- problem list contains a new condition that may contraindicate a long term drug or be caused by it
- blood tests are needed
- new illness has developed that may require drug dosages to be changed
- a different form of treatment is now indicated   [506]

Patients need information on how to reduce the risks of spread of infection when the diagnosis is concealed from carers or neighbours who help in emergencies   [610]

Never assume that written consent is the same as informed consent   [356]

Insurance company questions about AIDS risk need not be answered by GPs who may wish to record "Not practice policy to answer these questions. Refer to applicant"   [486]

How long has it been since this patient's control was assessed? Recall systems may be used for certain groups of patients who need long term follow up. How can this be organised? His repeat prescription card should indicate when he was last seen by the doctor and when he is due to be seen again (506).

Blood levels are needed to assess treatment and perhaps indicate levels of compliance. How can risk to the neighbour be reduced? (610)

This patient should not allow non-medical helpers to dress cuts or wounds resulting from fits. These should be dealt with by the patient himself until medical help can be obtained. He needs to be given dressings and shown how to apply first aid measures.

Case 81

A man aged 35 is gay and very anxious about AIDS. He requests an HIV test which was done and was negative. A few months later you were asked for an insurance report for which the patient has given signed consent to provide information. He indicates that he does not want to see the report before it is returned. A few weeks later he comes to see you and is very upset. He was refused an endowment insurance and was surprised to hear that the report disclosed that he was at risk of AIDS. This was the only fact in his medical history which seems likely to have led to the refusal. What is your response?

Patients give consent for the release of information without knowing what questions are being asked (356). This is not the same as informed consent where the patient knows the nature of the information to be disclosed. He could have been asked to make an appointment to ensure that he knew what questions were being asked (486).

> Patients need information on the medical, social, psychological, occupational, insurance, and mortgage implications of a positive HIV test before deciding whether to give informed consent for it to be done   [395]

> When counselling for HIV tests, a checklist of points should include the fact that, if records indicate a test was done, even if the result was negative, insurance may be refused   [597]

This problem could have been prevented by ensuring that counselling for the HIV test includes all the relevant implications of having this test recorded in the notes (395).

Counselling must always precede the decision to have an HIV test. A checklist is helpful to ensure all relevant points have been covered (597).

The patient may need some time to consider all the implications of having this test. Many districts have HIV counsellors. Would you refer patients for counselling or undertake this yourself? If it is done in the practice, the topics covered should be recorded in the patient's records.

Case 82

A man aged 39 was diagnosed as having AIDS when he developed pneumocystis pneumonia. He is now better and feels fit. He requests a certificate to return to work. He is a central sterile supply unit technician in the local hospital. What is your management?

> Patients may develop an illness that presents a possible occupational risk to others, and specialist advice may be needed before certifying patient fit for work   [614]

> HIV infected health workers must seek medical and occupational advice and those who perform or assist in exposure prone invasive procedures must cease such activities while seeking further advice on work practices that may need to be modified or restricted to protect patients
>
> (*Recommendations of expert advisory group on AIDS*, DoH, March 1994)   [757]

Should the GP certify this patient fit to return to work? Does his HIV status present a risk to others in view of the sort of work he does? Sterile precautions would be a normal procedure in such a job, and his risk of bleeding is no greater than anyone else's. However, there is a theoretical risk of contamination of sterile supplies and relevant guide-lines[1] should be reviewed before deciding what to do (614, 757).

132

An HIV infected health worker who has performed exposure prone invasive procedures while infected must cease these activities immediately and inform the local Director of Public Health (or in Scotland the Chief Administrative Medical Officer or CAMO) in confidence or request that a physician acting on his or her behalf should do so

(*Recommendations of expert advisory group on AIDS*, DoH, March 1994) [758]

Doctors who know that HIV infected health workers under their care have not sought or followed advice to modify their practices must inform the regulatory body as appropriate, and also the Director of Public Health (or in Scotland the Chief Administrative Medical Officer or CAMO) in confidence

(*Recommendations of expert advisory group on AIDS*, DoH, March 1994) [759]

All matters arising from and relating to the employment of HIV infected health workers should be coordinated through a consultant in occupational health medicine

(*Recommendations of expert advisory group on AIDS*, DoH, March 1994) [761]

The new Department of Health guidelines state that the patient must inform his or her employing authority (758).

What ought to be done if the patient refuses to discuss his HIV status with his health service employer? This will depend on the risk of infection to others and whether or not exposure prone invasive procedures are performed (759).

This patient gave consent to discuss his illness with the relevant consultant and his supervising manager. Who is the relevant consultant? (761)

Employers must make every effort to arrange suitable alternative work and retraining or, where appropriate, early retirement for HIV infected health workers

(*Recommendations of expert advisory group on AIDS*, DoH, March 1994)   [762]

All patients who have undergone an exposure prone invasive procedure where an HIV infected health worker was the main operator should be notified of this

(*Recommendations of expert advisory group on AIDS*, DoH, March 1994)   [760]

Employers have a duty to keep information on the health, including HIV status, of employees confidential and must not give information which would allow deductive disclosure; this duty does not end with the death of the worker

(*Recommendations of expert advisory group on AIDS*, DoH, March 1994)   [763]

- Formation of an early doctor–patient relationship when the patient was well
- Continuity of care for the patient from his own GP
- Reduction of pressure on hospital clinic appointments
- Better use of specialist skills
- Increase in GPs' confidence and competence in caring for patients with HIV infection through a structured protocol of care

It was decided that his work did not present a risk to others, and he returned to his normal job. If this patient was a surgeon, however, he would not have been able to return to invasive surgical procedures (762).

The risk to surgical patients is small but do they have a right to know about it? (760)

Issues of confidentiality have been clarified in the Department of Health's guidelines (763).

Employers may need to be reminded of the right of employees to confidentiality in such cases. This right continues to exist even after the health worker has died.

Shared care

Grun and Murray evaluated the use of shared care protocols for asymptomatic HIV positive male patients.[2] Patients were invited to participate and were asked if they would like their GP to share their care. Patients held a coop card containing a summary of the relevant medical history, a record of drugs prescribed, and a chart for completion at each consultation. Baseline investigations were done in the clinic and the GPs saw the patients every three months. An annual review was done at the hospital. The advantages are shown in the box.

People with HIV/AIDS are often articulate and well informed. They are usually the "experts" and the GP needs to remember this fact.

Conclusion

Some doctors are reluctant to accept people with HIV/AIDS as patients because their problems are so complex and time consuming. Yet it is from these very patients that we have the most to learn. They are a challenge and bring their own rewards.

1 AIDS/HIV infected health care workers: guidance on the management of infected health care workers. *Recommendations of the expert advisory group on AIDS*, London, Department of Health, March 1994 COI/HSSH J02-2302AR.
2 Grun L, Murray E. Shared care better for GPs and specialists. *BMJ* 1994;**308**:538.

17 Mental illness

Decisions about the management of patients with mental illness are often difficult to make. Many factors need to be considered and their assessment requires fine judgement.

Case 83

A woman aged 45 who is a supermarket manager has four children, is divorced, and now has a legal battle for custody of her children. Normally she copes well with stress and has no problems at work. She calls for a home visit and is now depressed, abusive, and suicidal. She feels hopeless and is very worried about the impending court case. She is not deluded or hallucinating and blocks every suggestion of help. "Doctors are useless, psychiatrists are fools, tablets are rubbish." She says "What is to stop me from killing myself?" She demands you do something to help. When asked why she called for a doctor, she says it was because her son aged 16 asked her to. What is your management?

This is a difficult problem because all offers of help are rejected. The doctor feels impotent, useless, and angry. What is the risk of self injury here? (51)

In assessing the probability of suicide risk factors include:

- intense feelings of hopelessness and worthlessness
- depression with marked sleep disturbance
- suicidal ideation or planning
- poor physical health or much pain
- living alone
- recent stress or loss
- males over 45
- substance abuse (alcohol or drugs or both)
- previous psychiatric illness or suicide attempt
- previous inpatient psychiatric treatment
- family history of mental illness, suicide, or alcoholism
- AIDS or HIV positive patients
- loss of mother by death or separation before age 12
- three or more children under age five years
- lack of either a close, caring relationship or a job

(the last three factors apply especially to women) [51]

Some patients may be at risk of self injury or injury to others and need urgent assessment by a GP, psychiatrist, and social worker to decide if there are indications for admission under section   [137]

In a suicidal patient who refuses all offers of help, a domiciliary psychiatric visit should be considered   [52]

Patients at risk of suicide need observation for 24 hours a day, and supervision of their treatment, until risk diminishes   [476]

In reactive depression, the management objectives are to prevent self injury, loss of job, and disability in patient and relatives   [129]

She is a single parent under great stress and seems quite desperate. Every option has been considered and rejected. Assessment of urgency may be critical (137). Remember that decisions made by doctors and patients are only relevant for the circumstances of the time. Today this patient's aggression and anger affect her ability to make rational decisions. What was unacceptable today may be acceptable tomorrow Some options are more acceptable when suggested by a consultant rather than a GP (52).

What is the most appropriate management of a rational but suicidal patient? You could reassess the next day, ask the psychiatrist or the community psychiatric nurse to visit, telephone for advice, contact the crisis intervention team, try to section her, or take no further action (476).

Decisions about this high risk patient should be shared with the psychiatrist. Although she refused to see a psychiatrist, he felt a domiciliary visit was appropriate. She allowed him in and talked to him for an hour. He managed to get her to accept a small dose of antidepressant drug. In treating such a patient, it is important to have clear management objectives (129).

The follow up management was shared between the GP and the psychiatrist. She made a good recovery.

Case 84

You are called to see a woman aged 27 who had a normal delivery two weeks previously. Five years ago she had an episode of hypomania which responded well to lithium. Three days ago the symptoms and signs of hypomania recurred. The psychiatrist was asked to do a domiciliary visit and he recommended lithium treatment. He suggested a follow up visit to his outpatient clinic in the local health centre. He asks if you agree with this management. What is your response?

Lithium is the treatment of choice, but how much of a risk does she represent to herself and the baby? She should not be left alone as there is always some risk to the baby in a mother with an acute mental illness. Her husband was able to stay home for a few days and was willing to supervise the treatment. He was told about possible complications and when to call the doctor. What other important factor must be considered at this time? (241)

> In the management of postpartum illness all decisions must be assessed in terms of effects on mother and baby [241]

Mother and baby must be considered as a single unit. Any decision about one will affect the other (221).

> In women with babies, selection of appropriate medication is affected by method of infant feeding and vice versa [221]

Before selecting an appropriate drug, the doctor must decide if it is contraindicated. Lithium should not be given to women who are breast feeding. The options are to select another drug or to change the method of feeding. In this case the mother agreed to change to bottle feeding.

It is important for doctors and patients to realise that breast feeding can be restarted if desired, once the drug is stopped. Few people realise that any woman will lactate if a baby suckles at the breast although it may take a day or so for milk to be produced. This was the secret known to the "wet nurse" of the middle ages. This fact should be remembered when a women regrets her initial decision to bottle feed.

Case 85

A doctor aged 29 presents with a two month history of agitation, anxiety, and depression. He is a medical registrar and these symptoms are interfering with his work. He is not deluded or hallucinating, and has no suicidal thoughts. He is happily married and has two young children. There are no obvious precipitating factors. He comes to see you for three consultations outside surgery times. You both feel that psychotherapy might be useful but initially a psychiatric referral seems appropriate. Until now he has continued to work but he says he can no longer cope. He thinks colleagues may suspect he looks depressed, but fears his career prospects will be harmed if he is known to have had a mental illness. He is due to see the psychiatrist in two days' time. He asks for a certificate for two weeks' sickness but does not want you to mention depression. What is your response?

> A mental illness may be suspected by relatives and work colleagues before a patient comes to the GP [419]

This patient is a colleague and it may be tempting to agree to his request and give him a certificate stating that he has a viral infection. He is asking you to lie about the cause of his illness. Would a more "acceptable" diagnosis be in the best interests of the patient? (419)

> The patient must identify the possible outcomes of a misleading certificate [420]

> If a patient is given a misleading certificate, the outcome may be that work colleagues may suspect worse problems, for example, AIDS, drug addiction, alcohol problems, or psychosis [421]

He says that his colleagues suspect that he is depressed. This is a common illness with a good prognosis (420). It is important to review the possible outcomes of agreeing to his request. What will colleagues think when they see a certificate stating "viral infection"? (421) Suspicions of worse problems would be more difficult to overcome if a false certificate were given (423).

> Most employers would be relieved to hear that patient has a mental illness that is readily treated, unlikely to recur, and will not adversely affect future occupation [423]

Another important factor to consider is that in rule 422. If the patient is no better in two weeks what would you then put on the certificate? Very few "viral" infections last longer than a week. This doctor, like any other patient, should be told that depression is one of the most common illnesses experienced by people in this country. It has a good prognosis but it may take a month before he is fit enough to return to work. He needs to consider the advantages of informing his consultant. Arrangements can be made to put in a locum and relieve the stress on his colleagues (424).

> Before deciding to issue a misleading certificate, consider the natural history of the patient's real condition [422]

> Consent to discuss an illness in confidence with a patient's employer may ensure adequate sickness replacement and more support on returning to work [424]

After thinking about these issues he agreed to allow the consultant to be told about his illness. He was very relieved to hear that it was just depression and not a psychotic illness. He was grateful to be told and suggested putting in a registrar locum for a month to allow adequate time for treatment to take effect. The patient made a good recovery and went on to a senior registrar's post a few months later.

A false certificate was given because he wished to have some confidentiality when it came to medical personnel and administrative staff. Would you have agreed to this unethical request?

Case 86

A new patient aged 30 has just moved into a women's refuge. She is eight months' pregnant and has schizophrenia which has been treated with haloperidol for the past year. She has three young children with her. She left her previous home because of violence from her partner. She wants to have the baby in a local hospital and asks if you can arrange this for her. She has her antenatal record from her previous hospital but left it in the hostel. What is your management at this time?

> It may be necessary to obtain urgent information about new or temporary patients from a previous GP, other hospitals, or Department of Social Services
> [594]

> A new or temporary patient may have children on the child protection register, and this possibility can only be considered in relation to their past or present problems   [657]

> For effective management of chronic disease, alcohol problems, and addiction, care needs to be shared; to do this, the responsibility and tasks of each person, including the patient, should be clearly identified and acceptable to all concerned   [286]

More information is needed about this patient but her records will take many weeks to arrive (594).

Information is needed about the whole family and not just the mother (657).

Her previous GP may be able to provide information about her medical and social problems. If there are case conference records these could be sent to you. Her social worker should be contacted to find out whether the local social services have been notified of this family. Good communication is essential to ensure continuity of care in such cases. The next person to contact is her psychiatrist. This might provide an up to date picture of her mental illness and its management.

She is eight months' pregnant and information is urgently needed to plan her care, based on relevant information from all concerned. Her care needs to be shared with the psychiatrist, obstetrician, GP, social worker, midwife, and perhaps the community psychiatric nurse (286).

There is a great danger that things become so fragmented that care is poorly coordinated. The GP is responsible for long term care and is well suited to ensure good communication between all concerned.

Case 87

A man aged 28 is a schizophrenic and always goes into hospital as a voluntary patient only to discharge himself 24–48 hours later. He is never properly treated and usually returns to the surgery hyperactive, paranoid, and very agitated. He asks to be admitted as a voluntary patient and you feel that you must comply. The parents are distraught and ask you to ensure that he is admitted without the ability to discharge himself so as to be certain that he gets the treatment he needs. He responds well once he gets injections of fluphenazine (Modecate) and then is able to return to work. What is your management?

Admission of a mentally ill patient under a short term section order can be converted by hospital staff into a 28 day order if necessary [139]

This patient usually accepts one or two injections and then stops all subsequent treatment. When he deteriorates he agrees to voluntary admission but knows he can refuse treatment and leave when he likes. Sectioning would ensure treatment could be given for a longer period of time (139).

Discussion between the GP and consultant may be the best way to overcome management problems and meet the patient's needs [438]

The hospital staff are reluctant to section a voluntary patient. This is understandable, but treatment can become impossible to administer (438). Discussing the problem with the psychiatrist helps to review the effects of this illness on the family. The management objectives include helping his distraught parents (331).

One problem may affect many people in a family who also need help and support [331]

This patient always responded dramatically to fluphenazine injections. This restores normal mental function and enables him to keep his job. Just before he becomes completely psychotic he would request an injection, but if this was not given immediately he would rapidly become irrational and refuse all further treatment. Follow up decisions are critical to effective long term care. It is essential that the patient continues treatment for long enough to produce a good remission (65, 67).

When patients with chronic mental illness relapse, it is important to distinguish between the objectives of crisis management and rehabilitation [65]

Follow up management of patients with mental illness should be jointly planned with the GP and psychiatric staff before discharge [67]

The immediate psychiatric discharge summary should indicate:

- dates of admission and discharge
- who referred patient to hospital: self, GP, community psychiatric nurse, social worker, psychiatrist, police, other
- type of admission
- diagnosis and initial management
- mental state on discharge
- who discharged patient: self or doctor
- accommodation on discharge: home, hostel, sheltered, other
- medication
- specific advice
- risk factors: lives alone, single parent, little family support, young children, divorced, recent bereavement, housing problems, social neglect, no fixed abode, multiple admissions, history of self injury, drug or alcohol problems, poor compliance, violence
- work prognosis
- follow up plans: who, what, how, where, when
- date of surgery appointment if follow up in general practice
- whether shared care record initiated   [663]

Roles and responsibilities for follow up will be clarified by joint planning before discharge. This should also include responsibility for follow up when he defaults from his appointment (663).

A pilot study of the use of an action oriented immediate psychiatric hospital discharge summary (as opposed to the final report written some weeks later) is described in a study that I undertook in 1991.[1]

If it is decided that the first injection after discharge should be given in the practice, a surgery appointment for the patient must be made before discharge. If this is done, and the patient does not attend, the notes will be there to remind the GP that this patient needs to be seen. If no appointment is made, the GP will not know that the patient has defaulted, and the whole cycle will recur.

- Community treatment is agreed with patient before discharge, and initiated by mental health team
- There is an identified key worker
- If a patient defaults on the agreement, the key worker calls an immediate case review
- The decision to readmit to hospital is based on existing criteria of the Mental Health Act
- There would be no additional powers to treat in the community

Mental health law

The recently introduced supervised discharge recommends the points in the box. These will have little effect other than to identify the responsibility of the "key worker." Supervised discharge orders may result in the allocation of scarce community resources towards the small group of patients to whom the orders are applied.

A recent conference organised by the Law Society, Mental Health Act Commission, and Institute of Psychiatry[2] highlighted the need for radical legal reform. It concluded that the law should be designed specifically for provision of care in both hospital and the community. It suggested that reform should be based on the principle of reciprocity.

"Patients' civil liberties may not be removed for the purposes of treatment if resources for that treatment are inadequate. Protection of society from nuisance or violence is insufficient reason for detention. Legal provision for compulsion of patients, whether in hospital or community, must be matched by specific rights to treatment. Psychiatric patients are distinguished from all others because their condition places them at risk of civil detention. Even if resources are inadequate to ensure specific rights to treatment for all NHS patients, they must be given to psychiatric patients."

Referral decisions

- Psychiatrist, psychologist
- Community psychiatric nurse
- Crisis intervention team
- Emergency outpatient clinic
- Psychiatric registrar in accident and emergency department
- Counsellor, social worker

It can be difficult to know to whom a patient with a mental illness should be referred. There are many specialists who might be able to help, including those in the box.

- Urgency, severity, risk to patient
- Family support, availability of other people
- Time of day, past history of illness or violence
- Previous involvement with patient
- Acceptability, previous treatment, and outcomes
- Local indications, guidelines, protocols
- Reason for referral, patient's and family's requests

The decision about referral will be determined by the factors in the box.

It is important that colleagues provide clear guidelines on what constitutes an appropriate or inappropriate referral. This is essential when care is shared. When a psychologist, community psychiatric nurse, or counsellor starts to work with the practice, it is useful to discuss how best to work together. Skills need to be recognised and the patients most likely to benefit should be identified. Patients should understand that the initial objective of referral is for assessment to identify the most appropriate form of treatment.

Purchasing services

Special problems may present to purchasers of services for mentally ill people. There may be a GP representative on a "focus commissioning group" which makes decisions about services to be purchased for the non-fund holding practices in the district.

Case 88

You are the GP representative on a focus commissioning group purchasing mental health services for a population of 1.4 million people. There is a discussion about the allocation of funds among the 30% fund holding practices and the rest of the practices in the area. The inner city population are nearly all served by non-budget holders. You are asked for suggestions about the basis for distributing this funding between the two types of practices. How do you respond to this request?

The relationship between markers of social deprivation and admission to psychiatric hospital is well established, and the use of such information in allocating resources has been strongly advocated. Kammerling and O'Connor have identified a sevenfold variation in the rates of people under 65 years of age admitted to psychiatric hospitals from small areas within a single district health authority.[3] This was far greater than the variation in any other specialty.

143

Ninety three per cent of this variation could be explained solely by the unemployment rates during the period of study. The unemployment rate in an area reflects its socio-economic status, and is a powerful indicator of the rates of serious mental illness in patients under 65 years of age who are likely to need treatment in hospital. This should be considered when allocating resources, particularly to fund holding practices. Failure to do so might cause considerable disadvantage to people living in areas of high unemployment.

This information is useful in trying to make a fair distribution of resources, especially as fund holding practices are often in districts where there is little social deprivation.

Case 89

You are the GP representative on a focus commissioning group for mental health services set up by the District Health Authority. There have been several complaints of sexual assaults on women in the mixed wards of a major provider unit. When brought to the attention of the ward staff it was usually dismissed as being part of the patients' delusions. Several patients have reported these assaults to the community health council and their representative has now presented a paper to the focus commissioning group expressing objections to mixed wards for severely disturbed mentally ill patients. What other options might be considered?

This focus commissioning group make important decisions about how the budget for mental health services for 1.4 million people is to be spent. It decides which tenders will be funded, and what other services ought to be provided in the community. When this problem was initially raised by the community health council representative, the managers discussed the issue with the providers. It was felt that the policy of mixed sex wards could not be changed. No other options were considered.

This is an example of a need perceived by patients but not shared by purchasers. Mixed wards are cheaper to run but are not acceptable to many female patients. Cost is not the only factor to be considered. The first question should be "how big a problem is this?" Hospital staff may not report such incidents and patients may be too frightened to do so. Should a questionnaire be sent to patients who have recently been discharged? Are there any reliable data from other districts? One option might be to admit male patients who represent a risk of violent behaviour to men only wards. A past history of violence to self or others is the best predictor of violent behaviour in hospital. Does the provider have a patients' advocacy group and, if so, what role does it play in such complaints?

The group should have considered options that are acceptable to the community health council's representative, and those responsible for taking action should be identified.

The GP representative was surprised that, at these meetings, no minutes were taken. It would be difficult to recall what was discussed and impossible to clarify disputes about decisions that were made. It was suggested that minutes should be kept and that an agenda for such meetings would be useful. Participants also requested the relevant papers in advance of such meetings.

Case 90

You are the GP representative on a focus commissioning group for mental health services set up by the District Health Authority. At this meeting the group is considering several competing proposals by different providers. A proposal has been presented by a provider unit for funds to train and employ two community psychiatric nurses to identify and manage adolescents with behavioural disturbances. These nurses would work alongside the consultant psychiatrists in the outpatient clinics. The Community Health Council and the purchasers have given priority to the unmet needs of this group of people. The committee seem to have reached agreement to provide funds for this project. What other factors need to be considered before making a final decision?

This proposal makes assumptions about the best place for such nurses to work. Should this service be provided in a psychiatric outpatient clinic or be community based? Most of the adolescents with behavioural problems are never referred to the outpatient clinic; they may present to GPs, social workers, or teachers whose school psychology service no longer exists. It would be more appropriate to place such skilled specialist nurses in the community. Perhaps the diabetic community nurse provides a model for such a group of patients. It was decided to support this proposal only if the nurses were to be employed to meet the needs in the community, rather than just care for patients seen in hospital clinics.

Case 91

You are the GP representative on a focus commissioning group for mental health services set up by the District Health Authority. A proposal is being discussed for a community mental health centre which would provide social support and also identify possible employment opportunities for mentally ill Afro-Caribbean patients. One of the managers feels that this is inappropriate because all mentally ill patients in the community, regardless of racial origin, should have access to this facility. You are asked for your opinion. What factors need to be considered before making a decision about this proposal?

- Policies regarding equity:
  —access
  —current levels of need and provision for these groups of patients
  —social support
- High risk groups
- Prevalence of illness
- Precedents
- Purchaser/provider priorities and goals

This can be an emotive issue and the most relevant factors that need to be considered include those in the box.

High risk antenatal patients receive care from consultant obstetricians which low risk groups may not receive. Patients at high risk of suicide receive closer follow up than other groups of depressed patients. Patients known to receive less skilled care and follow up may need more resources to achieve equity with other groups of patients.

Current statistics show that a higher proportion of Afro-Caribbean mentally ill patients end up in prison, compared to other ethnic groups who are more likely to receive hospital care. There is a greater proportion of Afro-Caribbean people unemployed compared to other groups, and the relationship between unemployment and serious mental illness needs to be considered. Yet the prevalence of serious mental illness in all ethnic groups is the same.[4]

What weight should be given to this information when considering the objections to this proposal? Ethical issues relating to equity (same treatment for same needs) seemed to carry less weight than information indicating greater needs and lower levels of provision for this group of patients. The proposal was accepted after discussing these issues.

Case 92

You are the GP representative on a focus commissioning group for mental health services set up by the District Health Authority. There are two groups of people who you feel have unmet needs. These include the needs of families looking after patients with schizophrenia, for respite care, and the needs of single mothers with mental illness. The purchasers have not identified these as priority groups and have no proposals from providers for services for these specific groups. There are many proposals from the psychiatrists in the local mental health units for other groups of patients who are less socially isolated. How should this issue be debated and what factors ought to be considered in deciding whose needs to meet?

How does the purchaser identify priorities and who participates in such decisions? Do purchasers and providers meet to try and agree on priority groups and services? The needs of these groups have been overlooked because no one saw fit to act as their advocates. What is the view of the Community Health Council? Does the GP represent an individual view, or the view of the local GP forum? (845, 847, 848.)

Rationing, setting priorities, and monitoring the implementation of guidelines should be a collaborative activity involving:

- FHSAs, purchasing authorities
- medical audit advisory groups, health professionals
- patient groups and those representing the poor, elderly people, those with learning difficulties, ethnic, and other minority groups [845]

When rationing resources to specific services, decisions need to be made about whether treatment, prevention, and community care services should receive equal or special priority [847]

When rationing resources should special groups, such as the young, the old, people with young children, and those whose illnesses are perceived as self inflicted, receive different priorities [848]

The District Health Authority should seek the views of voluntary organisations such as MIND, SANE and Newpin. Newpin is a valuable community resource for single parents. The purchasers indicated that this voluntary organisation was already meeting the needs of single parents with mental and social problems, and mentioned the very small "one off" grant of £5000 given to them last year. Since then, they have opened five new centres in south London and have been overwhelmed by the demand for help. It was decided to ask this organisation to submit a proposal for further support.

Purchasers have to identify their own priorities after consultation with relevant groups. In this process some groups may, however, be ignored. Flexibility is needed to be able to change priorities when vulnerable groups have been overlooked.

These problems highlight the advantages of having GP representation on such focus commissioning groups set up to share difficult decisions about services and priorities.

Conclusion

GPs must represent their patients and act as their advocates in discussions with purchasers and providers. It is an example of how much we care for patients with mental illness, and that care extends to decisions made by managers about what will be bought and sold in the market place.

1 Essex B, Doig R, Rosenthal J, Doherty J. The psychiatric discharge summary: a tool for management and audit. *Br J Gen Pract* 1991;**41**: 332–4.
2 Eastman N. Mental health law: civil liberties and the principle of reciprocity. *BMJ* 1994;**308**:43–5.
3 Kammerling RM, O'Connor S. Unemployment rate as predictor of rate of psychiatric admission. *BMJ* 1993;**307**:1536–7.
4 *Report on International pilot study of schizophrenia*, Geneva, World Health Organization, 1973.

18 Violence

The risk of violence is increased when a home visit is made to:

- a patient who has a past history of violence
- section a patient
- remove a possession
- remove a child from the family
- someone whose behaviour is unpredictable
- give unwelcome information
- someone under the influence of alcohol, drugs, or solvents
- a patient who is deluded or paranoid [840]

When visiting a patient where there is a risk of violence or aggression, consider being accompanied by a colleague or even the police, and clarify the roles and responsibilities beforehand [841]

In cases of violence in the home, the police can only assist if the patient is prepared to take legal action [443]

A court injunction may be obtained to try to prevent further acts of violence in the home [85]

Domestic violence often necessitates a joint consultation to assess needs, improve relationships, and prevent recurrence [659]

This is becoming an increasing problem facing doctors, nurses, and social workers. It can, however, often be predicted and the objectives should be to prevent violence wherever possible. The most powerful predictor of violent behaviour is a past history of violence to self or others. Information should always be sought about the past history when trying to assess the risk of violence. Other factors that increase the risk relate to the task that is being undertaken (840).

If there is a risk of violence, what precautions should be taken? (841) It may be safer to go with a colleague. Someone in the practice ought to know that you have gone on a visit where violence is a possibility. There should be a plan to telephone in within a specified period of time and, if this does not happen, staff must know what action to take.

Most acts of violence occur in the home, and police are reluctant to become involved in what seem to be domestic disputes (443). Women are most often the subjects of such violence and they need to know what options are available to prevent a recurrence (85).

Recently, some police stations have set up domestic violence units which are effective and acceptable to many women. If possible, the GP should try to consult with the perpetrator of violence within the home (659).

Alcohol and drugs often accompany violence and this may be the presentation of an underlying medical or social problem. Some mental illnesses increase the risk of violence. Some paranoid patients represent a possible risk of violence, although the prevalence of violence in schizophrenic individuals is no greater than in other groups of people in the community.

The Clunis Report[1] recommends that GPs should be informed of all aftercare plans, invited to attend aftercare meetings, and sent discharge summaries. Before removing a patient from the practice list, advice must be obtained from the local psychiatric team; if the patient is on the supervision register, the responsible medical officer must be informed and another GP willing to accept the patient should be identified.

Case 93

Your practice partner is doing his morning surgery. A patient has just left the room and he pressed the buzzer on the desk for the next patient. The door opens and in rushes a man with a large carving knife. He closes the door quietly and says "I'm going to kill you." When asked why he says "You know why." He does not move or say anything more. There is no panic button but an alarm signal was sent by continuously pressing the button for the next patient. You enter this room and recognise the patient who is a schizophrenic removed from the practice list three years previously. He was convinced that your partner had put the voices in his head that send him frightening messages. After talking to him for a few minutes, he finally hands over the knife. You leave the room to telephone for the police. When you return, you find the patient is holding another knife above your partner's neck. The police finally arrive and he hands over the second knife. They take him away to be sectioned. His GP telephones to say that she has just sectioned him for 28 days. He lives in a hostel near the health centre and had been receiving injections regularly at her surgery until seven months ago when the community psychiatric nurse decided that the injections should be given in your health centre. She said that he had been admitted with an overdose four months ago but had not been violent to her knowledge. The psychiatrist is on holiday. The community psychiatric nurse admitted knowing about his delusions but said that they were often getting threats from their patients. What further thoughts do you have about this episode?

A mentally ill patient whose paranoid delusions focus on a GP or any other member of the practice staff, or primary care team, should be removed from the list but the new GP should be informed of this risk   [654]

Abusive and violent patients can be removed from the list immediately   [892]

Doctors are responsible for informing colleagues about new patients if there is a risk of violence   [635]

The circumstances of violent behaviour are important in terms of prevention of recurrence   [658]

Every practice should have a written policy containing clear and concise guidelines for the management and prevention of violent or aggressive behaviour   [858]

This traumatic incident raises many isssues relating to prediction, prevention, management, and follow up. Three years ago this patient was removed from the practice list because the delusions were focused on one of the partners (654, 892).

The patient was living in a local hostel at the time, and his care worker registered him with another local GP (635). He had been living locally but had not attempted to see this partner for three years. This premeditated episode may have been precipitated by bringing him back to this health centre for treatment (658).

This traumatic episode could have been prevented. It was clear that the community psychiatric nurse knew about the delusions focused on your partner and yet he decided to bring the patient back to this health centre for treatment. Why was such a decision made when he had been receiving his regular medication with good compliance from the nurse in his own GP's surgery? There should be an enquiry into the circumstances of this decision. Who was responsible for deciding to move this patient back to this health centre? Are such decisions made by the nurse or is this the psychiatrist's responsibility? How do psychiatric staff assess the risk of violence in such patients? The lack of panic buttons made it difficult to alert staff to such a dangerous situation (858).

It was fortunate that there was an agreed signal for urgent help—the continuous use of the button summoning the next patient. This could, however, have precipitated a fatal assault. The procedure was for the receptionist to summon help from one of the male partners but not to enter the room herself.

Staff who have been subjected to violence or aggression need follow up support which includes:

- allowing the person to describe the event and talk about their feelings
- identification of the effects of the violence upon the victim
- allowing time to rebuild confidence
- identification of methods of prevention of recurrence
- review of practical issues, for example, insurance, compensation, sick leave, access to counselling, legal advice, etc
- consideration of the reallocation of duties on a temporary or permanent basis
- support of others involved in the incident
- recording the incident as per practice policy
- reporting the incident to the police
- analysing the incident to see whether it might have been predicted and prevented
- reassessing practice policies for reducing risk and protecting staff [859]

A doctor, nurse, or social worker must be warned immediately if a mentally ill patient's paranoid delusions focus specifically on him or her, as this represents a real risk of violence [652]

When such incidents happen further support is needed but rarely provided. Few doctors would consult their own GPs after such an incident (859).

Should support be provided by the partner's GP, the psychiatrist, or another partner in the practice? The need for follow up support is not well recognised. Doctors come off badly in such situations. People tend to be embarrassed to offer help to medical colleagues.

An irresponsible decision made by the nurse was compounded by failure to inform the doctor at risk about the new place of treatment. The roles and responsibilities of the nurse need to be reviewed. Knowing the background of this case, a unilateral decision to move this patient back to this health centre should not have been made without consultation with the psychiatrist (652).

The patient was admitted under section to a secure ward in a psychiatric hospital. However, after two weeks he was moved back to the local mental health unit. It was planned to discharge him within the next three weeks. What rights does the victim have to be told of his return to the local hospital and of his imminent discharge? Is this information confidential? This raises an ethical dilemma. Are there grounds for breaching confidentiality?

Where should the patient be sent on discharge? The psychiatrist felt that he ought to return to the same local hostel so that they could then "keep him under surveillance." This was far from reassuring news.

The Director of the Community Trust agreed to pay for panic buttons to be installed immediately. The patient returned to his previous hostel, stabbed another resident three times, and was sent to a secure unit.

Case 94

A woman aged 27 consults with a black eye and bruises. She has been assaulted by her partner. She says that this has happened twice before but she wants the injuries documented. She says that their relationship becomes violent when he drinks a lot. Usually things are alright. She would like a certificate to say that she needs a week off as she does not want to go to work looking like this. What is your management?

This patient's trauma is related to her partner's uncontrollable violence. It would be useful to try to see him alone or with her. The medical, social, and psychological impact of the problem on everyone in the family needs to be assessed. Plans can then be made to try and help the family and prevent further violence.

It is important to document the history and the specific injuries carefully as this case may come to court. Have her children ever been on the child protection register? (893) Such women are more at risk and the child protection register of this and other districts where they were recently living should be checked.[2] The risk of violence to children in the family is often overlooked. There is recent evidence to suggest that such children are in need of increased protection and the health visitor might be an appropriate person to visit and assess their needs.

> Mothers of children on the child protection register are more at risk of violence and assault than mothers not listed on the register, and children of women who have been assaulted are in need of increased protection [893]

Options

Effective management decisions depend on selecting the most appropriate options. An option menu can be a useful decision aid. Brathwaite[3] identifies a series of options for the management of a potentially violent situation.

1 Remove yourself from situation
2 Arrange to see the person at another time
3 Keep your voice calm and even
4 Do not shout
5 Make no sudden movements
6 Be polite and objective
7 Do not point at the aggressor
8 Try to control your own anxiety
9 Do not give a cigarette to a potential aggressor as it is a potential weapon
10 Try to distract before becoming involved
11 Break the process of "freezing"
12 Do not signal "victim"
13 Sit down
14 Establish eye contact but do not stare
15 Do not ignore the person
16 Give the person space, an exit, respect
17 Do not patronise
18 Remind the aggressor of past successes
19 Do not make ultimatums you cannot enforce
20 Do not stand by windows, particularly if the aggressor is now outside
21 Build on self esteem of the aggressor

continued

22 Practise the techniques outlined previously
23 Let colleagues know where you are going and when you intend to return if there is a risk of violence
24 Walk in a lighted area
25 Carry a personal alarm readily available
26 Do not take any undue risks
27 Have a policy on violence and use it
28 Take someone with you if:
   - person is unknown
   - person has a history of violence
   - there is a risk of violence and you are removing liberty or a possession
29 Call the police before rather than after an event
30 Determine a policy for dealing with people under the influence of drugs or alcohol
31 Plan potentially difficult encounters beforehand with a colleague

- list "risk" elements
- identify goal of visit or consultation
- review methods of defusing agressive behaviour
- record your movements and reporting back procedure

32 Installation of panic buttons in appropriate places
33 Light car parks and walkways wherever possible
34 Take threats seriously and do something about them
35 Anticipate high risk situations and plan interventions
36 After the incident do not assume it is over
37 Renegotiate the relationship
38 If you attend a self defence course go on refresher courses periodically
39 If people are fighting, call the police and remove others in your care from the area

40 Attend to needs of victim:
   - provide understanding, comfort, warmth
   - encourage victim to talk and share experience
   - provide someone "to take over"
   - counselling to overcome anger, insecurity, guilt, self blame, doubt
   - time to explore the incident and readjust
   - a clear choice about future contact with aggressor
   - information about compensation, insurance, legal systems
   - to be supported, not interrogated
41 Implement strategies for prevention of recurrence
42 Schedule time to discuss the incident

Conclusion

These options form a useful basis for planning how practice staff can prevent, anticipate, and manage a potentially violent situation.

Prediction of risk is important and, before discharge from a psychiatric hospital, the risk of violence must be assessed. Past behaviour, the situation in which any violence occurred, and the nature of any delusions are the best predictors of future risk of violence.[4]

1 *Report of the inquiry into the care and treatment of Christopher Clunis*, London, HMSO, 1994.

2 Ward L, Shepherd J, Emond A. Relationship between adult victims of assault and children at risk of abuse. *BMJ* 1993;**306**:1101–2.
3 Brathwaite R. *Violence: understanding, intervention and prevention*, Oxford, Radcliffe Professional Press, 1992.
4 Groves T. Psychiatrists must assess risk of violence. *BMJ* 1994;**308**:224–5.

19 Communicating decisions

Management decisions need to be communicated to all involved in care. The inability to do this causes considerable morbidity and sometimes mortality. It is more accurate to talk about a failure of people rather than of communication.

Case 95

A man aged 35 with progressive hydrocephalus but normal intellect is admitted to hospital with a severe chest infection. On the ward round a student asks why a shunt cannot be put in. The consultant says that it would be too dangerous to insert one at this age. Student says "then there is little hope." The patient immediately telephones his father to say that he wants to come home. He is very upset and tearful. He tells him about this conversation and says that he has been written off. His father comes to tell you that this has just happened. "What should be done, doctor?"

> The GPs role includes communication of anxieties of patients and relatives to hospital staff [287]

> The ward sister is often the best person to clarify management, deal with communication problems, and provide information about progress and plans of hospital patients [463]

Such insensitive comments cause great distress. How can the GP help this patient? (287) Many problems concerning hospital management are brought to the GP who may need to liaise with hospital staff (463).

The ward sister will be able to bring this episode to the notice of the relevant doctors and students. She is on the spot and would be able to reassure the patient. If you cannot get hold of the sister, would you ask the houseman, the registrar, or the consultant?

The objective is to clarify the facts. You have only heard a third hand report of what was said, and it may not be accurate. The consultant needs to know how distressed this patient is. With good communication this problem can be resolved, and more awareness may prevent a recurrence on future ward rounds.

Case 96

A man aged 45 has an inoperable carcinoma of the bowel. He has been discharged from hospital after a laparotomy which showed so many secondary deposits that a colostomy could not be done. He is now totally obstructed. He is being looked after at home. He is on a liquid diet and receives drugs from a syringe driver which is providing good pain control. He came to London nine months ago because of a new job. The family have no support in London, however, and all their relatives and friends are in Manchester. You visit and they tell you that they have decided to return to Manchester in two weeks' time. He is very weak and his condition is deteriorating. "Do you think we have made the right decision, doctor?"

The decision of whether or not to go to Manchester is a personal one. The GP may, however, help in decisions about when and how to travel. Important factors are estimation of life expectancy and the rate at which he is deteriorating. He is now very weak and his condition is rapidly worsening. His life expectancy is measured in weeks. The patient needs to consider these facts before deciding when to go (455).

> Patients and doctors should have access to all relevant information before making irreversible decisions [455]

This is a delicate matter to discuss. It was suggested that, having decided to go, it might be better to do so as soon as possible. This would enable him to enjoy the company of his relatives and friends for a longer period. It was better to travel when he was feeling stronger than in two weeks' time when he might feel weaker. They decided to pack the house up later, and to go that weekend.

He will need immediate nursing and medical care as soon as he arrives in Manchester. This must be organised before departure. His new GP must be contacted by telephone and told of the situation. The patient should be given a letter outlining the current problems and medication. He should also be given the contents of his records. The district nurse needs to contact her colleagues in Manchester to inform them of the time of his expected arrival, and current nursing needs. The plan was for the family to contact the new GP as soon as they arrived in Manchester. Good communication is essential if effective continuity of care is to be achieved in such a case.

Case 97

A woman aged 27 was discharged from hospital a week ago. She had an intrauterine death at 36 weeks and was admitted for induction of stillbirth. She is very distressed because the community midwife visited yesterday and left a note to say that it was very important to come to the antenatal clinic at this stage of pregnancy. She left an appointment for her to attend that week. What is your management?

> Those who need to be informed about deaths and stillbirths may include doctors, nurses, health visitors, midwives, and appointment and transport staff, and records should indicate who has been told [630]

> In cases of unexpected death or stillbirth, a home visit should be done to provide bereavement counselling, support, and to re-establish confidence [105]

> In cases of unexpected death or stillbirth, recent patient management should be reviewed to identify preventable factors [563]

There has been a most unfortunate lack of communication here (630).

Why was the midwife not informed of this stillbirth? (105) A home visit is always appreciated after an unexpected death or stillbirth. It provides an opportunity for an uninterrupted talk with both parents. Such a visit had not been done in this case (563).

Were there any risk factors or any early warning signs such as decreased fetal movements? Was there delay in seeking advice and if so why did this occur? Patients often fail to recognise the importance of decreased fetal movements, and this may account for the delay in seeking help. None of these questions should be asked directly as it is important to avoid making the parents feel guilty.

Communication with district nurses

GPs and district nurses work as a team and it is vital that they agree on the methods of communication to be used. An understanding of each others' work patterns and stresses can help to alleviate misunderstanding and reduce frustration.

District nurses visit on average eight to ten patients a day; it might be necessary to discuss five of these with a GP each day. In a group practice with six doctors and three nurses, communication can be difficult. Slipping into the surgery between patients is unsatisfactory for all concerned. A special time should be set aside each week to discuss problems and ensure effective shared care.

District nursing notes are now being left in the patient's home as patient held records. The use of the GP sheet could greatly improve communication, especially as more than one doctor might be visiting.

The need for reattendance

In a survey of 300 consultations, doctors and patients were questioned about the need for reattendance. GPs judged that 74% needed to reattend. There was a low coefficient of agreement, however, between patients' and doctors' views on whether reattendance had been recommended. Control of doctor initiated consultations is limited by clinical considerations and the difficulty of accurately communicating the doctor's advice on reattendance to the patient.[1]

Action oriented discharge summaries

Continuity of care depends on good communication between hospital and GP. The final inpatient summary often takes some weeks to arrive. An appropriately designed initial discharge summary could contain enough information to dispense with the final report received weeks after discharge. For psychiatric patients, immediate information is essential. GPs have identified the information needed on discharge of mentally ill patients.[2]

- Dates of admission and discharge
- Who referred patient to hospital: self, GP, community psychiatric nurse, social worker, psychiatrist, police
- Type of admission, diagnosis, and initial management
- Mental state on discharge
- Who discharged patient: self or doctor
- Accommodation on discharge: home, hostel, sheltered, other
- Medication, specific advice given
- Risk factors: lives alone, single parent, little family support, young children, divorced, recent bereavement, housing problems, social neglect, no fixed abode, multiple admissions, history of self injury, drug or alcohol problems, poor compliance, violence
- Work prognosis, follow up plans: who, what, how, where, when
- Date of surgery appointment if follow up in general practice
- Whether shared care record initiated

The immediate psychiatric discharge summary should indicate the points in the box. Action oriented discharge summaries, which clarify the roles and responsibilities after discharge from acute psychiatric units, have been used to great effect. It provides essential information that ensures effective continuity of care and follow up. How many providers use such a summary? GPs should persuade purchasers of the need to build such basic minimal standards of information transfer into their contracts with providers. Without such criteria, continuity of care will always be suboptimal.

1 Armstrong D, Glanville T, Bailey N, O'Keefe G. Doctor initiated consultations: a study of communication between general practitioners and patients about the need for reattendance. *Br J Gen Pract* 1990; **40**:241–2.
2 Essex B, Doig R, Rosenthal J, Doherty J. The psychiatric discharge summary: a tool for management and audit. *Br J Gen Pract* 1991;**41**: 332–4.

20 Requests

Many requests are made by patients and it can be difficult to decide how to handle them. They range from the routine to the unethical, from the predictable to the unimaginable.

Case 98

Your receptionist is telephoned at 1.30 p.m. by a woman who says that her mother has had a bad headache since last night and she is most anxious that a doctor comes to visit. Her own doctor refuses to visit but has diagnosed sinusitis and left a prescription at the surgery. The daughter is very worried and telephoned the Family Health Service Authority who said her doctor must visit, but he again refused. She asks if you would go even though you are not her doctor. She lives 2 miles from the surgery but is not on the telephone. What do you do?

You could select one of the options in the box.

> Give advice
>
> Try to contact her GP
>
> Ask her to come to the surgery if possible
>
> Tell her to go to the accident and emergency department
>
> Do an emergency home visit
>
> Suggest she gets a 999 ambulance

> If a visit is requested by someone who is not your patient because his or her doctor refused or was not available, it is your responsibility to:
> - assess the need
> - act appropriately and
> - inform patient's GP   [553]

The daughter said that her mother was too ill to come to the surgery. She has tried hard to obtain urgent help. The differential diagnosis includes serious conditions such as a subarachnoid haemorrhage and severe hypertension (553). These factors affected the decision to visit.

The patient had a severe headache and neck stiffness. The diagnosis of a subarachnoid haemorrhage was confirmed by lumbar puncture after admission to hospital. The notes were written on an emergency treatment form and the reason for the visit was recorded as "own general practitioner refused to visit." It is important to keep a record of clinical findings and management on a separate continuation sheet as there is no room for these observations on the claim form.

Case 99

A woman aged 61 requests a medical certificate stating that she has retired on medical grounds. Although she does not get much pension from her UK job, she can obtain one from Germany where she worked for 12 years before coming to the UK. To do so she must have your statement that she retired on medical grounds. Her records show only one visit during the year for an anxiety state which seems to have settled. She says she gave up work because she could not cope with the stress. What do you do?

The records show little evidence to support her request. There is no reason to disbelieve the patient when she says she had to retire on medical grounds. Many patients experience severe disability as a result of depression or stress without coming to the doctor (554).

> Certification can be based on the patient's statement and not only on recorded observations   [554]

At such times it is not easy to decide what to do. Judgement must determine the best course of action. The doctor's support could make a great deal of difference to this patient's life.

Case 100

An Iranian man aged 32, recent UK citizen, has just joined the practice. He is afraid that his parents' lives are at risk if they stay in Iran; this was during the early stage of the new Islamic regime. His father is a lawyer but is no longer allowed to practise. He asks you to write a letter to the embassy saying that he is undergoing investigations for a potentially life threatening illness and requesting permission for his parents to visit on compassionate grounds. What do you do?

> If a life can be saved by behaviour that is professionally unethical, the doctor must decide what takes priority   [290]

Would you lie to get this man's parents out of Iran? Are there ever circumstances when a doctor should behave unethically? (290)

A doctor is supposed to save lives whenever possible, and a failure to do so will weigh heavily on the conscience. There may be a conflict between the duty to save lives and the duty to behave ethically (289, 291).

What priority should be given to ethical principles in this case, when the cost of preserving ethical principles could be someone else's life? Which is easier to live with? If such a letter were written the conditions under which this was done would have to be clarified. Total confidentiality is essential and no one should know that such a letter was written. It would be embarrassing to find that a demand has been created. It would also be prudent to state that no gifts can be accepted.

Every possible scenario should be considered before deciding what to do in such an unusual case. It is naive to imagine that doctors always behave ethically. It may be in a patient's interest that, on rare occasions, other priorities take preference. In this case the need to save life may be considered to have a greater priority. It may be helpful to discuss options with a wise colleague. When this case was discussed with a group of trainees, no doctor was prepared to lie. One wonders what action would be taken in the privacy of their own surgeries.

> When doctor's and patient's values conflict, consider whether duty to save life has priority over doctor's right to protect own ethical values [289]

> Before deciding to take a risk, assess all possible outcomes for doctor, patient, relatives, and others who may be involved [291]

Case 101

It is this man's second marriage and he has had a failed reversal of his vasectomy. The couple went to a private hospital for artificial insemination by donor and his wife has just had a live healthy baby. The hospital where she had the baby was not told about the artificial insemination. She now asks if the letter about the artificial insemination could be removed from her practice records. They never want the baby to know that the husband is not his biological father. They are desperately anxious about this, and ask you to give them this letter. Do you agree to their request?

Knowledge that the mother had
artificial insemination may be
very relevant to a child if the
natural (as opposed to the
biological) father develops a
genetic disease, and this should
be remembered if patients
request removal of information
about artificial insemination by
donor (AID) from the records
[632]

People often ask the doctor to do things without considering all the possible consequences, and the outcomes of this action should be discussed (632).

The parents should consider whether their child would ever need this information in later life? This couple may feel differently when they have had a chance to accept this baby as their own. Counselling may help to identify the real fears and anxieties that surround this request.

Case 102

The parents of a child with Down's syndrome come to request referral for facial cosmetic surgery which is now available on the NHS in some centres. They say it will make the child more acceptable to others and less conspicuous. The father asks if you think that this is a reasonable request. What is your response?

Value judgements affect decisions made by patients and doctors, and it is difficult to be objective. The GP's personal views about the use of NHS resources for cosmetic surgery are not relevant here. The father has asked if this is a reasonable request. There seems to be some doubt in his mind. It is worth exploring his feelings about this option before responding to this question. This case seems to be about acceptability of one child by other children. Perhaps it is also about the acceptability of this child by her parents? Is surgery the only option to increasing social acceptance or are there less painful solutions? (390)

Psychological assessment of the
patient and careful review of the
reasons for a request may be
needed before reaching decisions
about certain kinds of
treatments, for example,
cosmetic surgery   [390]

A psychological assessment might enable the relevant issues to be explored before making such an important decision. The management objective should be to identify the parents' feelings about their child and her acceptability by other people. This decision is very difficult for the parents, and there are ethical and social factors that need to be considered (389).

Psychological, ethical, and social
dilemmas surrounding a
particular management option
ought to be considered before
referral   [389]

The parents accepted referral to a psychologist but still requested referral to the plastic surgeon.

Case 103

A mother brings her child aged nine months as an emergency at 6.30 p.m. You saw the child for the first time on a home visit two days previously. They have only just registered with the practice. At that time he had a fever with no abnormal findings. You advised paracetamol syrup and to review if still febrile in two days. There are no new symptoms but he still has an intermittent temperature. There is no rash, and ears and throat are normal, abdomen soft, and chest clear. There is no neck stiffness or enlarged glands. You explain to the mother that this is a viral infection and that she is doing the right thing. He will improve and that her request for antibiotics is not appropriate as viral infections do not respond to antibiotics. She seems rather unhappy but does not argue. Your receptionist comes to tell you that she has now asked to see one of your partners and she wants to know what she ought to do. What is your response?

The initial reaction may be one of anger. A competent history and examination have been done, and time has been spent explaining to the mother what the problem seems to be. The surgery is very busy and it is very likely that she will be given similar advice by the other partners. The options are in the box.

- Offer her an appointment for another doctor tomorrow morning?
- Discuss this with your partner and get her fitted in that evening?
- Send her to the accident and emergency department?
- See her again yourself to try and reassure her once more?

Consider the consequences of each option. If her request is refused she might request a night visit. If you use a deputising service she may get the antibiotics that you do not feel are indicated. She is asking for a second opinion and it may be advantageous to agree to this now. If the child turns out to develop meningitis or pneumonia it will be useful to have the agreement of two doctors about the findings that evening (891).

If a patient is unhappy with your management, the problem is acute, and the receptionist is asked if another doctor can be seen during that surgery session, this might:

- provide a second opinion to support your management
- reduce the patient's anxiety
- identify something you had missed
- prevent a night visit
- prevent a complaint should a serious illness develop subsequently   [891]

This is a strategy for the prevention of complaints or allegations of negligence. It is also important to remember that a colleague might diagnose something that was missed.

Case 104

A woman aged 70 comes to discuss her concerns surrounding the death of her sister aged 84. She was put on
a life support machine and remained on it for three weeks.
It was something that she would have abhorred and it
upset all the relatives. She realises that she might have a
stroke and be unconscious and unable to express her
wishes. She requests that you record her request to with-
hold all life support in such circumstances. What other
considerations are relevant?

Competent patients may give
advance directives that are
instructions about which
treatments they wish to be given
or which withheld should they
subsequently lose the capacity to
give consent because of physical
illness or mental incapacity, and
such directives are legally
binding   [804]

Advance directives ensure that the wishes of a competent
patient are considered when informed consent can no
longer be obtained (804).

Patients need help to draft advance directives, and they
also need an explanation about the illness and its possible
treatments (805). Such directives should be considered
legal documents and the records must indicate clearly that
these have been drawn up (806).

Advance directives indicating
consent for treatment should be
drafted by the patient with
guidance and counselling from a
doctor about:

- natural history of disease

- treatment options

- risks and advantages of such a
  document

and should be reviewed by
patients at least once every five
years   [805]

Advance directives in which
consent or wishes are clearly
established and applicable to the
circumstances are as legally
binding as any current decision
made by a competent patient[1]
                           [806]

When treatment has been initiated before the discovery of advance directives that are contrary to the patient's specified wishes, it should be discontinued and if a proxy decision maker has been nominated this person's opinion should also be sought[2]

[807]

It is the patient's responsibility to ensure that the existence of an advance directive is known to those who may be asked to comply with it[2]

[812]

What should be done if treatment has started before the existence of advance directives has been discovered? (807)

The patient must tell all relevant people about the existence of such directives (812).

Remember that advance directives cannot be made to cover future treatment of a mental disorder.

Case 105

Your partner tells you about a young woman aged 18 who came to ask for a letter to help her obtain accommodation from the local authority. She explained about her mother's neglect and cruelty, and was clearly distressed in trying to describe this. Your partner felt that this information ought to be taken into account by the housing authority when considering the daughter's request. The mother is also a patient in the practice. He wrote the letter. Some weeks later he receives a letter from a solicitor acting on behalf of the girl's mother. It talks about litigation for defamation. He is quite distressed and now regrets writing the letter. He asks you whether you would have written it or not. What is your response?

To prevent litigation for defamation based on unsubstantiated allegations, great care must be taken about what is written about others and to whom the words are conveyed

[766]

One can understand the desire to help this patient but did the letter make an unsubstantiated allegation or not? (766)

Much depends upon how the letter was phrased. Did it state that this was an allegation made by the daughter? Could it have been written in a way that did not make unsubstantiated allegations? At this stage, the goals are to obtain urgent expert advice and to provide support for the partner whose distress is understandable.

Case 106

A woman aged 32 is dying of carcinomatosis from cancer of the colon. Her husband was working in Vienna when she became ill and a laparotomy was done there. She was found to have inoperable carcinoma of the colon. They decided to return home to London for her terminal illness. She is receiving home care from you, the district nurses, hospice team, and relatives. She has two boys aged two years and 10 months. It is now 6 p.m. on Saturday and her husband telephones to say that she has just died. When you visit to confirm the death he says that the Austrian surgeon mentioned that at laparotomy he saw some polyps. Before death she was deeply jaundiced and the abdomen was full of tumour and ascites. The husband asks if there is any point in having a postmortem examination to exclude familial polyposis. What is your response?

> If uncertain about the need for or potential value of a postmortem examination, seek expert advice from a medical specialist, geneticist, or pathologist [648]

> A postmortem examination should be considered even if there is only a small possibility of identifying a cause of death that may be familial and may necessitate screening of other relatives [633]

This request was made as you leave the house. The death has been extremely traumatic for all concerned. It is not very likely that a postmortem examination would be informative as she had such extensive carcinomatosis, but there has been no time to consider this decision which could have profound effects on this family (648). There is uncertainty about the need for a postmortem examination, and it seems wise to obtain expert advice. The case was discussed with a gastroenterologist who advised that a postmortem examination ought to be done (633).

The postmortem examination was arranged by contacting the local hospital pathologist. It could have been done by the coroner's pathologist but the hospital specialist was excellent and this was thought to be the best option.

Case 107

A woman aged 26 comes to see you. She wants a paternity test done as she is not certain about the father of her son aged three years. She had an affair which ended a few weeks before she became pregnant. She thinks that the father is likely to be her husband but would like to be certain. Her husband knew about the affair but believes that the child is his. What is your response?

This is a difficult situation and all the relevant factors must be carefully considered. Patients often think that such a request can be done on a routine basis with the consent of a parent or assumed parent. Would it be in the child's interest to have this test done? The child's interests must be considered because he is the most vulnerable party. The test could have profound effects on the attitude of those caring for him. It also has implications for the presumed father who is unaware that the child's paternity is in doubt.

Such testing cannot be carried out simply at the request of the adult parties involved, but is subject to strict regulation. The Home Office issues guidance on this subject and regularly nominates a very limited list of doctors authorised to carry out paternity tests. This request conceals her anxieties which ought to be explored before deciding on the advisability of the test. Many requests made by patients are precipitated by unresolved anxiety and guilt. The doctor's perception of the problem will be clarified by exploring the reasons behind such requests.

Case 108

A friend telephones you at 7 p.m. just after evening surgery on Thursday 30 December. He is not your patient. He says that his brother-in-law who is Spanish and lives in Madrid is very ill with cancer of the prostate. He has bone secondaries and his doctor feels he needs a course of goserelin (Zoladex) injections. This drug is very difficult to obtain in Spain and a friend has come to the UK with a private prescription written by his Spanish doctor. The family are able and willing to pay for 12 of these injections. Their local pharmacist has obtained them but the prescription needs to be endorsed by a British doctor. He says that his friend is returning to Spain in two days' time. He asks if you would be prepared to endorse the prescription if he brought it round after morning surgery tomorrow. What is your response?

The options for action are in the box.

- Agree to endorse the prescription
- Refuse to do so and risk upsetting a long standing friendship
- Get the Spanish doctor to purchase the drug from UK suppliers
- Try another pharmacist to see if they would accept the Spanish prescription without an endorsement
- Obtain further advice

This request was for a drug which was in the *British National Formulary*. It costs £500 for eight injections and it is indicated for carcinomatosis secondary to prostatic cancer. It seemed a reasonable request but all possible outcomes need to be considered. The Medical Defence Society was contacted the following morning. Their expert pointed out that by endorsing such a prescription the doctor is assuming clinical responsibility for a patient who has not been seen. This includes responsibility for any serious treatment complications. The General Medical Council would take a very dim view of any decision to endorse such a prescription, and the position would be indefensible. Reluctantly this decision was explained to the friend and other options such as buying directly from the company were considered.

The following week a patient comes to see you, saying that you saw her mother who was visiting from Trinidad last year. She had hypoparathyroidism following a thyroidectomy and needed alfacalcidol tablets. She is going to visit her mother and says these tablets cannot be obtained in Trinidad. She would like to take a supply of this medication for her mother who is under regular medical supervison. She asks if you would be kind enough to write a private prescription for her to take with her. How should the doctor respond to this request in view of the above comments?

This patient had been seen as a temporary resident a year ago and at that time this medication was prescribed. It can be a life saving treatment and these facts affected the decision to give this patient a private prescription for her mother. She was asked to obtain a written report from the doctor in Trinidad stating the diagnosis and that this treatment would be taken under medical supervision. In such a case, care is shared by the prescribing doctor who depends on the medical opinion of the examining doctor.

Case 109

A woman aged 36 consults because she has read about a test which shows whether a person will develop Alzheimer's disease. Her mother has this condition and she wants to know if she is also likely to develop it. She brings the newspaper article[3] which discusses the test and mentions that the science journal *Nature* is advertising apoprotein E test kits. She would like to do a test on herself and her children, and asks if you could do the test without her having to buy the kit. What is your management?

This is a difficult problem, and it is always wise to ask the patient to bring the article to read. This summarised a paper in *Nature* in which French scientists described the test for the gene called *apoE*. This can indicate whether a person has a good life expectancy. The apoprotein E test can, however, also reveal with 90% accuracy if an individual will develop Alzheimer's disease by the age of 65. The article also reports the comments of Professor James Scott.

> Anyone offered a test for a genetic disease must understand that it is voluntary and be told:
>
> - about the disease they may have
> - what can be done to treat it
> - how reliable the test is
> - how a positive result might affect their family   [897]

He wrote to *Nature* to condemn the adverts and kits. He said "guidelines to protect the individual from injudicious genetic testing are not clearly established." The editor of *Nature* is directly responsible for carrying such adverts knowing that it is unethical to offer patients a screening test for an incurable and untreatable genetic disease (897).

This patient needs to be counselled about the test and its implications for herself and her children. She should know about the implications of 90% accuracy as well as the possibility of false positive results. She also needs to consider how her life would alter if the result were positive. The clinical geneticist was telephoned to discuss this test, and he offered to see the patient for counselling about the issues surrounding it.

At present there are no laws to address this problem, in spite of constant warnings that people may be pressurised by insurance companies or employers to take genetic tests. This is an issue that the profession should take up with the Government.

Case 110

You see a man aged 42 who has been seeing your partner over the last few weeks. He initially complained of intermittent fever and cough. His chest was clear and he was reassured that this was a viral infection. He returned several times with vague aches and pains and had been treated for an anxiety state in the past. Your partner has written that "this patient is obsessed with minor psychosomatic symptoms and is neurotic about his health. His symptoms relate to his chronic anxiety." You find nothing abnormal on clinical examination but do a full blood count, an ESR, and a chest radiograph. This shows a high ESR and the chest radiograph shows a mass in hilar regions. The diagnosis could be malignancy or a lymphoma and he is admitted for further investigation. A few weeks later there is a letter from the FHSA inviting your partner to comment on a letter of complaint about his management of this patient. He is embarrassed by the comments he wrote about this man, and would like to rewrite his notes. This would involve you rewriting your own notes on another sheet. What is your response to this request?

It can be difficult to know what to do in such circumstances. There is a conflict of interest between ethical issues and the desire to help a partner. This is a comment about the symptoms and is not a record of clinical observations themselves. There is no request to add or delete any clinical information. Would you agree to this request or seek advice from your medical defence organisation? If you agreed to rewrite your records on a new continuation sheet would you photocopy the originals first or not?

Assume that you agree to this request, and when you see his "amended" record you find that it is a much fuller account of clinical symptoms and negative findings than the original contained. What would you now do? It is possible that both doctors could be found to have falsified a critically important document. A Questioned Documents Forensic Expert can show with surprising accuracy whether or not entries are contemporaneous.[4] It is never worth altering clinical records.

1 Re T [1992] 4 All ER 649; Airdale NHS Trust v Bland [1993] 1 All ER 859.
2 *Medical ethics today: Its practice and philosophy*, London, BMJ publishing group, 1993:163, 178.
3 Mckie R. Test for Alzheimer's gene may wreck lives. *Observer* 2 Jan. 1994.
4 Schutte A, Gilberthorpe D. Altering records – beware of the pitfalls. *Journal of Medical Defence Union* 1994;1:6–7.

21 Mistakes

- Wrong identification of problems or diagnosis
- Important task not done, for example, follow up
- Failure to educate patient
- Roles and responsibilities not defined
- Lack of knowledge
- Lack of skill
- Failure to communicate relevant information
- Relevant factors not considered
- Failure to follow up patient
- Management option not considered
- Inappropriate assumptions made
- Failure to resolve uncertainty
- Important decision not made
- Decisions made in the wrong order
- Right tasks done in the wrong order

Identification of the cause of mistakes is as important as making a differential diagnosis of an observation or symptom
[756]

The GP is responsible for follow up of patients who default or did not attend, unless someone else has agreed to take on this task
[26]

Doctors are often in error, but seldom in doubt. Students and trainees are expected to learn from their mistakes, but teachers must ensure that the right lessons are learned. A differential diagnosis of the aetiology of errors is shown in the box.

It is important to learn from our mistakes to prevent them from recurring.

Case 111

A man aged 52 complains of upper abdominal pain and slight weight loss for six weeks. A barium meal is ordered because he did not want an endoscopy. He was asked to come back one week after radiography. Six months later he returns with severe upper abdominal pain and weight loss. On examination he looks anaemic and a mass is felt in the upper abdomen. The barium meal report in the notes says that he has an ulcer which could be malignant, and suggests an urgent endoscopy. The report has been signed and the box marked "see doctor" has been ticked. This indicates that an appointment would have been made for him to see you. He is immediately admitted for investigation. Do you do anything else?

A mistake has been made and this needs to be investigated (756).

Who is responsible for the failure to follow up this patient? (26)

> Good organisation ensures that investigation results and letters are seen and appropriate action is taken when the doctor is away, or the patient defaults or did not attend for follow up [12]

> To prevent problems in patients with appointments who did not attend or defaulted, records should be examined to decide if follow up is needed [11]

> • Receptionists ensuring that the notes of patients who did not attend are reviewed by the relevant doctor before refiling
> • Attaching the abnormal result to the front of the notes without filing them to ensure that it is not overlooked if the patient does not attend

The report showed that the "see doctor" box was ticked. The receptionist would have telephoned or written to ask him to see the doctor. The old appointment sheets would show if he had made an appointment. If he did not attend, what further action should have been taken? (12)

How can the doctor ensure appropriate action is taken in such circumstances? (11)

If the records had been examined, the reason for the appointment would have been apparent. He might have been asked to make another appointment or a home visit could have been done. On this occasion the GP was called out to an emergency visit and the last three appointments were distributed to partners with the exception of this patient because he did not keep his appointment. The receptionist did not mention this and the record was filed.

In general practice, poor organisation or inadequate procedures are responsible for more serious errors than wrong diagnoses. The goal is to prevent a recurrence. A new procedure is needed to provide a safety net for the follow up of patients who do not keep their appointments. The options should be discussed with partners and the practice manager. They include those in the box.

This patient assumed that the result was normal otherwise the doctor would have notified him. What should the patient be told about this error? Consideration of the patient's rights will affect subsequent management.

Case 112

A man aged 42 called for a night visit because of cough and fever. He told the deputising doctor that he was allergic to penicillin. The doctor prescribed ampicillin and assures him that this would be safe. Three days later he developed a rash, ulceration of lips, palate, gums, and severe exfoliative skin rash. He remains at home for 10 days and recovers slowly. He wants a certificate to return to work. What is your management?

It is every doctor's responsibility to try and prevent a colleague from repeating the same serious mistake [38]

The patient has the right to be informed if the illness was drug induced, even if no questions have been asked [542]

Legally the GP is responsible for the mistakes of the deputising doctor, unless he or she is also a principal in general practice [39]

The management objective is to prevent a recurrence of this serious error (38).

Should this case be discussed with the deputising doctor? Should the patient be told the rash was the result of being given penicillin? (542) It is unwise to be too critical of colleagues and patients are often reassured by an offer to discuss the outcome with the doctor concerned to ensure that it does not happen again. It is useful to discuss the management of this sort of case with your medical defence organisation (39).

This policy is currently under review. The deputising doctor was contacted and he accepted responsibility for the error. He had not realised that penicillin sensitivity included ampicillin. The patient did not make a formal complaint.

Case 113

A woman aged 46 has been discharged from hospital in a full length plaster cast after a road accident in which she fractured her femur. You are called because she has now developed severe calf pain in the plastered leg. She also complains of pain in the ankle which is swollen and she cannot bear weight on it. This had been mentioned to the hospital doctor but a radiograph was never done. You refer her back to hospital to exclude a deep vein thrombosis and request a radiograph of the ankle. This was done and she was told in hospital that it was normal. After several weeks she requests a legal report and you telephone the hospital to get the radiography report. You are told that there was a fracture of that ankle. What is your management now?

All investigation results and letters should be signed by a doctor before being filed [372]

Before responsibility for alleged mistakes, mismanagement, unprofessional conduct, or compensation can be identified, the facts from all concerned must be identified directly [408]

Fractures are easily missed, and the doctor who initially saw the film may have thought it was normal. However, the radiologist reported that a fracture was present. Does the hospital have a system for ensuring that action has been taken when abnormal investigations are reported? (372) If there is no such system, there should be; if there is, it may not be followed. This needs to be clarified with the hospital staff (408).

Responsibility for finding out results of hospital investigations rests with the GP [369]

The general practice records should be reviewed to ensure that a hospital report or letter about this fracture was not overlooked. Although the GP requested the radiograph in the referral letter, no attempt was made to obtain the result (369).

Those of us who work in the NHS soon learn never to assume that no news is good news.

Case 114

You are consulted by a lady aged 30 who has Hodgkin's disease. This was first diagnosed seven years previously, and she was treated with radiotherapy, chemotherapy, and splenectomy. She did well and has had no recurrence. She now presents with gangrene of the tips of her fingers caused by recent severe pneumococcal septicaemia. This was treated in the local hospital for the last six weeks. Doctors told her that she should have been taking prophylactic penicillin since the splenectomy. She now asks for a repeat prescription card for penicillin. She wants to know why she had not been put on long term penicillin and what she ought to do about this omission. The family live in poor circumstances and her husband has recently been made redundant. What is your response?

Before responsibility for alleged mistakes, mismanagement, unprofessional conduct, or compensation can be identified, the facts from all concerned must be identified directly [408]

Is it relevant to discuss compensation at this time? (408)

There are two possibilities. One is that prophylactic penicillin was needed, and the other is that, at that time, the evidence for its use was not conclusive. If the evidence was good enough for long term antibiotics, was she given the relevant information? (411)

It is the patient's right to be given information on risk of surgical complications both short and long term, and how these can be diagnosed or prevented [411]

Who was responsible for informing this patient about the need for long term penicillin? (321)

Identify whether instructions were ever given by hospital staff to GP or patient about long term care and prevention of complications [321]

176

If the hospital state that long term treatment is indicated, unless otherwise stated, it is the GP's responsibility to ensure that this is provided [409]

When patient requests information about past or present treatment, this may be best provided by the doctor who initiated it [410]

Patients have the right to discuss questions relating to their management with the hospital consultant [322]

If evidence of effectiveness of prophylactic treatment is equivocal, decisions must be based on risk of event, its potential seriousness, and the side effects, cost, and acceptability of preventive treatment [412]

Patients who have had a splenectomy must be:

- counselled about the risk of infection and its prevention
- immunised against *Haemophilus influenzae* b, pneumococcal, and meningococcal infections
- provided with long term prophylaxis (amoxycillin)
- given an information card to help identify early signs of sepsis and take appropriate action
- given amoxycillin for self treatment of early signs of infection[1] [896]

The GP is responsible for her long term care. There may be a letter in her notes explaining the need for long term penicillin (409). This was not mentioned in any of the hospital letters. She is still under follow up in the lymphoma clinic and she wants to know why she was not put on penicillin (410).

It would be helpful if she could discuss her past management with the consultant who initially treated her for this illness. This is not passing the buck (322).

The case was discussed with the specialist, who said that seven years ago the evidence did not seem good enough to justify prophylactic penicillin after splenectomy. This was why it was not given. He was happy to explore this issue with the patient (412).

She felt better after talking to the consultant and realised that her confidence was not misplaced. She would have liked, however, to have been told about this risk before she had the operation. She wanted a chance to share the decision about the need for long term antibiotics, in view of the risk of serious infection.

Clinical practice should be based on best available evidence at the time of treatment. This was seven years ago. The evidence now favours prophylactic antibiotic treatment and immunisation (896).

If new information becomes available and policies change, how can such patients be recalled? This procedural problem may be worth discussing with the surgical directorate.

Case 115

You visit a woman aged 84 who lives alone and needs meals on wheels. She also asks for an ambulance to be organised to take her to the next outpatient appointment. You ask one of your receptionists to organise these services. Three weeks later you visit and discover that the transport did not arrive and there have been no meals on wheels. What do you do?

> The aetiology of a serious administrative or clerical error must be identified to prevent recurrence [350]

> A receptionist who is asked to organise a service for a patient must record that this has been done in the records [364]

In a large practice with many receptionists it can be difficult to remember who was asked to organise these services. It may not be possible to find out what has happened (350).

Whose fault is it that these things were not done? Is there a fail safe way of knowing if this request was made? It helps to record in the notes the name of the receptionist to whom this task was delegated (364). She or he should record that the relevant people were contacted. If this was done, then responsibility for failure to provide the services must lie elsewhere.

Case 116

A boy aged 16 had a neuroblastoma of the spinal cord which was treated with surgery, radiation, and chemotherapy 10 years previously. It was not possible to remove all the tumour but he has kept well since then. He has now developed hard bilateral supraclavicular glands. Four months ago he saw the trainee for a persistent cough and a radiograph showed a widening of the mediastinum. The report suggested urgent further radiology. The last entry by trainee says "to discuss with radiologist." The trainee left the practice three months ago. The patient's mother is very anxious because his cough is much worse and he is losing weight. What is your management?

> The aetiology of a serious administrative or clerical error must be identified to prevent recurrence [350]

A serious administrative or organisational error seems to have occurred (350).

Perhaps the trainee did talk to the radiologist. Maybe there was an agreement that further tests would be done but these were not organised. A letter may have been sent but not received. The notes should indicate whether the radiologist was contacted. Decisions made about further investigations should also have been recorded. If the trainee was not taught to do this, the trainer must share responsibility for the lack of information. A telephone call to the trainee established that no contact had been made with the radiologist. It seems that the notes had been filed before action could be taken (38).

> It is every doctor's responsibility to try and prevent a colleague from repeating the same serious mistake [38]

This might have been prevented if an action sticker had been clipped onto the front of the notes. This case should be discussed at a practice meeting. The trainer must ensure that trainees know how to prevent such an organisational error.

Case 117

A woman aged 39 presents with a fungating growth of the cervix and is immediately admitted to hospital. The growth is inoperable. You are following her up at home and she knows she has cancer. She has three children under the age of 14 years. The notes show that she had a cervical smear done five months before this presentation which was reported as normal. You and the district nurses visit regularly. What relevant factors affect the management of this patient?

Every test will have false negative and false positive results [61]

Malignancy following soon after a negative screening test raises the possibility of a false negative result, and necessitates an expert reassessment of the tissue initially examined; the GP may have to ensure that this is done [498]

A false negative or false positive investigation or screening test resulting from incompetence, ignorance, or negligence may have serious consequences for the patient, and such errors necessitate a review of the person's previous work [497]

Do management objectives just relate to the terminal illness or are there wider issues to consider? (61) Was the smear test done five months previously really normal? (498)

The pathologist was asked to review the slide. He telephoned to say that the slide was full of malignant cells and was unequivocally abnormal. This was a gross error on the part of the technician who examined and reported on it.

General practice cares for individuals, and also for risk groups within the practice population. The goals include prediction and prevention, as well as treatment. Concerns relate to other patients whose slides were examined and reported to be negative by the same technician (497).

Is it safe to assume that a review of the technician's work was done? Who is responsible for finding out? Other patients in the practice may have had smears examined by this technician. It is therefore the GP's responsibility to find out what steps have been taken to identify other false negatives. There are no safe assumptions when it comes to medical practice.

The histopathology consultant was telephoned to discuss this concern. He said that the technician had worked in the department for six months and had screened 2500 slides. He did not have enough skilled staff to cope with the present workload and said it was not feasible to review these slides. Much as he would like to, there were no funds to employ extra staff to do this work. Even if funds could be found, skilled technicians were scarce. He was asked if there was a hospital protocol for dealing with this sort of error. Similar errors have occurred in other districts. One might have expected that a policy on how to deal with them already existed. The consultant was not, however, aware of such a protocol.

What rights do patients have when errors of this sort arise? What responsibilities do health authorities have to their populations who have been screened by a negligent technician? If there is agreement that all the slides examined by this technician should be reviewed, should the pathology department or the Regional Health Authority (RHA) provide the necessary extra resources? The RHA might be able and willing to allocate special funds for this purpose. If this were not feasible, then perhaps the work could be divided between other departments in the region.

This pathologist has made a decision which could have profound effects on the health of many patients in your practice. The initial negligence is compounded if no attempt is made to obtain the extra resources needed to identify other false negatives. The pathologist was asked to inform the Regional Health Authority of this error and ask for the extra resources needed to review this technician's work. He said he would consider this suggestion.

When asked what had happened to the technician he said that she had moved to a similar post in another district. He admitted that he gave a reference which did not mention this error. This technician needed to be retrained under close supervision before being allowed to continue this sort of work. Serious errors of judgement seem to have been made. There are now doubts about the ability of this consultant to do what seems necessary in this situation.

By communication via the Local Medical Committee, the GP can try to ensure that hospital staff take appropriate action when problems arise in relation to screening, laboratory, or other hospital services   [541]

The goal is to prevent anxiety and distress to other patients in the district. The authority responsible for the district screening services should deal with this problem. The Local Medical Committee has GP representation (541). This option should be considered when discussion with relevant people has failed to resolve the problem. It is always helpful to discuss problems with the secretary of the Local Medical Committee who advised that a letter be sent to the chair person to alert the committee to the problem. The matter was then referred to the Director of Service Development and Public Health.

A few weeks later the Director sent a letter saying that the matter had been looked into in detail. Extra staff had been brought in to review the 2500 slides. A new quality assurance post had been created and the laboratory staffing problems were being dealt with. The authority now employing this technician was also alerted to the problem. This was a reassuring outcome which would not have occurred had the official channels of communication been ignored.

Should this patient be told of this error? She had never asked about the previous "normal" cervical test. She is now very ill and weak. Should the GP tell her about the mistake? Under these circumstances decisions are difficult to make and there is great uncertainty about what to do and how to do it (142).

Advice can be obtained from partners, ethical experts, the BMA, and medical defence organisations (533).

The great difficulties of informing a terminally ill patient about this error do not override the right of the patient and her family to be told. They have a right to compensation when negligence has been acknowledged. This patient was told there had been an error and she was asked if she wanted the matter pursued for her, but she declined. The family were also told of the screening error. They decided not to make a complaint against the health authority.

> When uncertain about the diagnosis or management of a potentially serious problem get urgent expert advice   [142]

> A patient has the right to be informed about a false negative or false positive result, especially if caused by incompetence or negligence   [533]

Case 118

A woman aged 42 is visited because she has developed severe upper right sided abdominal pain. You do not have her notes with you but she says she had undergone ultrasonography three months previously and was told at the time that she had a gallstone. She has had no recurrence of pain until now. You treat her for cholecystitis and explain that the stone needs to be removed. The next day you see, to your surprise, that the report on the ultrasonography in her notes states that the gallbladder was normal and there were no gallstones. What is your management now?

Discrepancies between what patients say that they were told and information provided in hospital letters or investigation reports need to be clarified by direct discussion with relevant staff [735]

Either she was misinformed or the report is wrong (735).

It is always safer to discuss such cases with the radiologist. The ultrasonogram did show a gallstone and this was a reporting error.

Case 119

A man aged 18 is seen by the practice nurse in the travel clinic. He is going to Zimbabwe and needs antimalarial advice as well as immunisation. The appropriate immunisations were given, and the nurse looked up the antimalarial recommendations for Zimbabwe. He was prescribed mefloquine. She wrote this out on a private prescription and got a doctor to sign it. A few days later the patient's mother telephones to say that the label on the bottle states that this drug should not be taken if the patient has convulsions or epilepsy. She reminds you that her son has epilepsy. What is your management?

The responsibility for prescribing rests with the GP. In practices where the nurse runs a "travel" clinic, however, she will look up the countries being visited, and will check this against current recommendations for antimalarial therapy. This may be part of the protocol which has been drawn up for this work. A travel clinic protocol should, however, also include the contraindications to antimalarial therapy. It was revised to include this important information. In future the nurse would refer such a patient back to the GP to discuss alternative therapies.

Conclusion

Any task based on judgement is fallible and errors will always occur. One of the strengths of a group practice is that partners pick up each other's mistakes and can correct the error before serious harm occurs and prevent a recurrence of the same mistake. The factors in the box enable us to learn from mistakes.

These cases highlight some of the more common errors in daily practice, many of which can be prevented by improved communication and organisation. Most serious mistakes occur because of poor administration and organisation rather than lack of diagnostic or clinical skills. The willingness to discuss one's own mistakes with partners, nurses, receptionists, and the practice manager helps everyone to learn from them. If doctors can admit their mistakes, others will also feel able to do so. It is very important to offer an apology to the patient when a mistake has been made. This is the sound advice that the Medical Defence Union offers to its members.[2]

- Good communication
- Ability to accept criticism
- Continuing professional education
- A forum within the practice where cases can be discussed
- Awareness that sometimes it is better to discuss an error with the individual concerned and not present it to everyone
- A trusting and non-threatening atmosphere

1 Flegg PJ. Long term management after splenectomy: national guidelines, please (letter). *BMJ* 1994;**308**:131.
2 Morrison MCT. A question of risk? (Letter.) *Journal of the Medical Defence Union* 1994;**10**:23–4.

IV Organisation

22 Practice staff

GPs employ staff and delegate many decisions to receptionists and practice managers. The role of employer will be new to many doctors and some of the issues surrounding these two tasks are analysed in this chapter.

Delegation to receptionist

What decisions are within the receptionists' competence to make? Should a receptionist decide whether a patient can be fitted into a booked surgery as an "emergency" or is this a decision the doctor should make? Most doctors would not be able to screen the large number of patients who feel that they need to be seen that day even when there are no appointments. This task is often delegated to the receptionist. Is it left to "common sense" or is any training given?

Who decides if a request for a visit is accepted or not? Is this task delegated to the receptionist or does the doctor screen the visit requests? Is the receptionist expected to identify the urgency of visit requests and, if so, are guidelines provided? Receptionists may have to make a decision on the situations in the box.

- A request for a visit is accepted
- A request for an urgent appointment is accepted
- A prescription can be accepted over the telephone
- A visit is urgent or not
- A telephone call should be put through to the doctor during surgery

The GP is responsible for deciding what tasks to delegate to receptionists. A clear job description helps to identify tasks that are to be delegated and competency based training can then be provided.

Staff employment

GPs are employers and need to know about employment law, employees' rights, and employers' responsibilities. The following cases illustrate some of the employment problems that present to GPs. The solutions presented relate to legislation in force in 1993–4.

Case 120

You employ eight part time receptionists, three of whom are your patients. The others feel that you are providing much better care than their own GPs and ask if you would take them on as patients. What is your reaction?

When patients are employed to work in the practice there may be a conflict of roles for the GP [392]

It may seem difficult to refuse as three of them are registered with the practice. They were, however, patients before they were employed as receptionists (392).

The doctor may have a conflict of interest when a receptionist becomes ill. Concern for the health of the receptionist may conflict with the need to get her or him back to work as soon as possible. If a receptionist has to be disciplined or dismissed, this could have implications for her or his health and might make it difficult to be objective about medical management (393).

Employing patients may have implications for patient confidentiality [393]

Receptionists will have access to their own records and the implications of this need to be considered. They will also see the letters and reports of other receptionists. Confidentiality would be better if they were registered with another practice.

Case 121

Your cleaner gives in her notice. She tells the practice manager that she wants a change. Later in the week, the caretaker says that she left because the practice nurse asked her to clean the speculums before they were put in the steriliser and she did not feel that this was her job. How do you handle this problem?

Job descriptions clarify the roles and responsibilities of everyone employed by the practice, as well as all members of the primary care team [726]

This sounds like an unprofessional approach on the part of the nurse. You cannot be sure, however, that this is really what happened. Before making allegations of unprofessional conduct the facts must be identified directly from the nurse. If she acknowledged that she asked the cleaner to do this task, the job description should be reviewed (726).

The nurse's job description should clearly state that she is responsible for ensuring that safe infection control measures are taken. This is the basis for a discussion about roles and responsibilities.

Case 122

A receptionist has been employed in your practice for five years. Her hours are 8 a.m. to 11 a.m., Monday to Friday. Since being a member of the practice staff she has been late many times. She has been counselled and warned. Last time she was half an hour late, she failed to offer a reasonable explanation for her lateness. You dismiss her with pay in lieu of notice. This morning you receive a notice from the Office of Industrial Tribunal that she has lodged a claim for unfair dismissal. What is your defence?

Does this receptionist come into the category of staff who are entitled to claim unfair dismissal? (737) Her age is not stated but could be relevant (739).

> Staff who are dismissed have the right to claim unfair dismissal if they have been employed for 16 hours a week for over five years, unless the dismissal is for an inadmissible reason such as sex, race, marital status, pregnancy, and childbirth   [737]

> Staff over 60 but under 65 have the right to claim unfair dismissal unless the practice has established a definite policy of retirement at 60 years of age   [739]

To defend a staff claim of unfair dismissal you need to demonstrate that:

- the practice has a disciplinary procedure
- your employee knew of the procedure and how it operated
- it was included or referred to in the written employment contract
- your actions followed all the rules and the sequential steps of the procedure
- you kept a written record of actions   [738]

The practice disciplinary procedure should specify that any breach of patient confidentiality is a very serious offence which normally leads to dismissal of staff   [740]

Staff over 60 but under 65 have the right to claim unfair dismissal unless the practice has established a definite policy of retirement at 60 years of age
[739]

She has been employed for 16 hours a week for over five years. She satisfies the basic qualifying conditions to complain of unfair dismissal. In your defence you would need to show an industrial tribunal that basic criteria were met (738).

The practice manager must ensure that the disciplinary procedure has been updated and is incorporated in the employment contracts of reception and clerical staff.

Case 123

A receptionist aged 62 has been a member of the practice staff for six years. She works 12 hours a week and while she was in the reception area she told a patient, Mrs Roberts, that another patient, Mrs Thomas, had just received long awaited confirmation of her pregnancy. Mrs Roberts met Mr Thomas on her way home and congratulated him on his good news. Unfortunately, this was the first news he had received about his wife's pregnancy. Although he was delighted he nevertheless complained to the practice manager about the breach of confidentiality. You immediately dismiss this receptionist for this behaviour and do not allow any further discussion of this incident. Two weeks later you receive notification that she is making a claim for unfair dismissal. How would you defend your actions?

Should breach of confidentiality be listed as grounds for dismissal? (740)

The practice manager should ensure that a breach of confidentiality is recorded as grounds for dismissal in the disciplinary procedure. This receptionist is over 60, and is not eligible to receive a state pension (739).

Practice staff need to be trained to recognise the importance of patient confidentiality and to work in ways that ensure that a breach of confidentiality is prevented   [741]

A disciplinary procedure should allow employees to explain their side of the story and, if it does not happen, a claim for unfair dismissal may be upheld   [742]

If a serious disciplinary offence is believed to have occurred, which would justify summary dismissal, the employee should be suspended on full pay while an investigation is conducted, to prevent a subsequent claim for unfair dismissal   [743]

She remains eligible to complain of unfair dismissal until she is 65. Staff need to be trained to ensure that confidentiality is maintained. What kind of training should be given and who should be responsible for ensuring that it is provided? (741)

The induction and training procedures should ensure that all staff know that the practice attaches the highest priority to patient confidentiality. Case studies of examples where confidentiality has been breached are useful for staff training. Confidentiality has been breached in this case so what possibility is there that she might succeed in her claim for unfair dismissal? (742)

The disciplinary procedure was not followed because she was not allowed to give her side of the story. This failure could lead to the dismissal being found unfair (743). Had the procedure in rule 743 been followed, this employee would have had no grounds for a claim of unfair dismissal.

Case 124

Your practice manager of 10 years' standing to date has only undertaken supervision of practice staff recruitment, and holiday and rota arrangements. In the light of recent contractual changes the partners have decided that it is necessary to upgrade the position of the practice manager. In particular you wish her to operate a computerised system which implements the new health promotion bands. She is reluctant to assume these new tasks and points out that these are not part of her job description. How should this problem be resolved?

The practice manager's job description, which is part of her employment contract, needs to be changed (744).

Changes in practice may necessitate the practice manager taking on new tasks which need to be:

- outlined in a revised job description which is part of the employment contract
- explained and agreed to
- incorporated in an appropriate training programme
- monitored until new skills are acquired   [744]

The first task is to explain why the change is necessary, and then seek her agreement in principle to the new tasks. If she agrees, she must receive adequate training and encouragement to develop these new skills. When she has become competent to operate the new computer system, there should be no further issues that need to be addressed. If she either declines the new work or is found to be incapable of doing it, she may have to be made redundant.

Case 125

You were recently interviewing for the position of practice receptionist. Five white and one Afro-Caribbean applicants were interviewed. You appointed one of the white candidates. You have just received notification that the Afro-Caribbean applicant is claiming that she has been discriminated against on the grounds of race. You believe that this claim is quite unjustified as this practice staff vacancy was filled by the most suitable applicant. How do you start to construct your defence and how might you prevent such a claim in the future?

> Practice staff recruitment and selection procedures must be designed to avoid any direct or indirect discrimination on grounds of colour, race, nationality (including citizenship), ethnic, or national origins [746]

Your defence will need to show that your selection procedures were designed to avoid discrimination (746).

Evidence of the recruitment procedure should always be kept (745). A written record is essential to defend a charge of discrimination.

> A written record of staff recruitment procedures should be kept to satisfy an industrial tribunal that racial or any other form of illegal discrimination has not occurred [745]

Case 126

You have a receptionist aged 35 who has not worked for eight months because of depression. She had previously worked for eight years for 35 hours per week and was considered to be a good worker. You are the senior partner in the practice and her GP. At the practice meeting it is decided that this practice staff position needs to be filled permanently as soon as possible, and you want to dismiss her on the grounds of ill health. How would you proceed?

> Before dismissal of an employee on grounds of sickness or ill health you should have:
> - considered the possibility of redeployment in less stressful work
> - obtained an independent medical opinion on the likelihood of her becoming fit for work again [750]

She has worked for at least 16 hours a week for at least two years and is therefore eligible to complain of unfair dismissal (750).

The first decision is whether alternative employment can be found for her in the practice. There should be a meeting with the practice manager to discuss this option. Minutes should be kept to show that alternative possibilities were reviewed.

The second decision is about the possibility of her becoming fit for work. Here an independent medical opinion is essential. Failure to do these two things will justify a claim of unfair dismissal.

Case 127

A member of the practice staff has been employed for the past nine months working 15 hours a week. She becomes pregnant and informs you that in a month's time she will start her 18 weeks' statutory maternity leave, 11 weeks before the baby is due. She also tells you that she intends to return to her post as receptionist on a full time basis after her 18 weeks' leave. You think this is impractical and inform her that after careful consideration the practice has decided that it does not wish her to return. What problems do you face?

Before making this decision it would be wise to review her legal rights (747).

If you were uncertain, expert advice should have been obtained from the BMA. No action should be taken before a careful review of the legal position is made. Could this problem have been predicted when she was first employed? What does her contract say about maternity leave? She is not being allowed to return and in effect this decision amounts to her dismissal. It could be interpreted as an unfair dismissal on the grounds of pregnancy/childbirth, which could be seen as discriminatory on grounds of sex. The new universal maternity right of 14 weeks' unpaid leave helps to clarify this issue.

> A pregnant employee has the right:
> - not to be dismissed on grounds of pregnancy
> - to return to her previous job after 40 weeks' maternity leave if she has worked for at least 16 hours a week for two years (or eight hours a week for five years)
> - to receive statutory maternity pay if she has at least 26 weeks' previous employment
> - to 14 weeks' unpaid maternity leave [747]

Case 128

You are informed by the Family Health Service Authority that the reimbursement for practice staff may well fall below the current 70% level and you are reconsidering all staff contracts. You intend to continue to employ the practice nurse on a series of one year fixed term contracts to avoid having to make redundancy payments. Are there risks in adopting this approach?

In a staff employment dispute, fixed term contracts may be regarded as continuous employment for the purpose of protection under employment legislation, unless the employee explicitly forgoes the right to claim redundancy compensation [748]

Employers who try to avoid the effects of employment legislation in this way are making a wrong assumption (748).

It is unlikely that an employee would give up the right to claim redundancy compensation. Any changes in your staff contract should be discussed with an expert to ensure that all the implications have been considered.

Case 129

You have a local authority nurse attached to your practice. He has created difficulties for some time. His attendance record and time-keeping are poor. In particular, there are long periods of protracted sickness which are not satisfactorily accounted for. His overall effect on other staff is to lower their morale. How do you manage this problem?

Problems arising with work performance of staff, for example, nurses or health visitors, attached but not employed by the practice should be made known to, and are the responsibility of, the manager of the employing authority [749]

The nurse is employed by the District Health Authority. Because you are not his employer, the action you can take is quite limited. Any disciplinary action has to be initiated by his employer (749).

This nurse's manager should be informed of these difficulties and asked to take the necessary steps to resolve them. Ultimately the practice could request that the attachment be ended. There may, however, be a risk of not getting a replacement, and leaving your practice without a nurse.

Case 130

Working relationships among your practice staff have reached breaking point. A senior receptionist has always had a somewhat difficult personality, but now the problem has reached the stage where none of the other staff will talk to her, and even you and your partners are finding it increasingly difficult to hold a normal conversation. She carries out her work properly so you cannot find any obvious grounds for dismissal. Everyone feels that if she is not dismissed soon you are in danger of losing your other staff. What is your management?

Breakdown in working relationships between members of practice staff are grounds for fair dismissal and it is important to adhere to the practice disciplinary procedure [751]

Fortunately there are grounds for dismissal if there is a breakdown in working relationships. In this case there seem to be good grounds for dismissal (751).

This is a common problem. Unsociable behaviour of this kind is often allowed to persist because no attempt is made to correct it. Annual staff appraisals provide an opportunity to help a receptionist to recognise such problems and to identify ways of dealing with them. If you decide to take disciplinary action which is likely to lead to dismissal, the practice disciplinary procedure must be carefully followed.

Case 131

One of your practice staff has a domineering and forthright manner. Some patients find this receptionist intimidating. Although she is good at protecting the doctors from patients, her manner has caused problems on several occasions. Patients have complained that she asks what is wrong with them in front of other patients waiting in the reception area. What is your management?

Practice staff whose attitude or behaviour is not acceptable need to be:

- informed of the problem
- told what change of behaviour is needed
- offered further training
- appraised regularly to monitor performance [752]

Although this problem has been evident for a long time, no action has been taken to deal with it. This receptionist is doing her job in a style that she has been allowed to believe is acceptable. No one has the courage to tell her otherwise. The longer this difficult task is postponed, the more difficult it becomes. She has to understand the effect her behaviour has on others and on her work performance. If you have a practice manager this should be her or his task (752).

Why has the problem been allowed to continue for so long? This issue should be discussed with the practice manager. Other concerns include the lack of confidentiality in the reception area and the management of patients' complaints.

If this problem had been dealt with as soon as it was identified, staff appraisal could be used to identify if performance had improved. The fact that this has been allowed to continue implies a lack of policy about confidentiality and the management of complaints.

Case 132

Most of the applicants for receptionist jobs in your practice are married women. Although it can be safely assumed that older applicants who already have children are unlikely to become pregnant again, younger applicants who have no children can present difficulties in a small practice if they become pregnant. To avoid these staff problems you have always asked applicants at the interview about their family plans. This has caused no problems until recently, when an applicant pointed out that your question was discriminatory. This has left the partners a little confused and anxious. It seemed reasonable to try to avoid problems of staff turnover and maternity leave if at all possible. You are interviewing for more staff next week. Will you ask this question again?

To ask any applicant for a job about his or her plans for family rearing is discriminatory (753).

Good practice management involves avoiding discrimination at all times. Any individual is eligible to complain of discriminatory recruitment procedures, irrespective of whether he or she has actually applied for your job vacancy.

> To ask a job applicant, male or female, at a staff interview about plans for family rearing is discriminatory on grounds of sex, and risks action being taken under anti-discriminatory laws
> [753]

Case 133

A frequent source of friction in the practice is the procedure for notifying annual leave. Every year the same difficulty occurs. All the reception staff want to take the same period of time off for annual holidays and occasional leave days. This is because they all have school age children and want to take their leave during school holidays. Your present system of approving leave encourages staff to rush through their leave requests as soon as the leave year starts. This is unsatisfactory and does not please anyone. What is your management of this problem?

Decisions about introducing changes must be made after consultation with all the staff (754).

By discussing the problem with the staff it may be possible to agree on a fair and equitable system for allotting annual leave. Everyone should recognise the need to resolve this

> Allocation of holiday leave should be made by a system that is fair, equitable, and agreed by all concerned; it might include:
> - giving priority of choice according to seniority
> - introducing a rota which enables each employee in turn to have the first choice of leave dates   [754]

problem in a way that allows the practice to run effectively during school holidays. The solution has to be seen to be fair by all employees. In turn, staff should be encouraged to adopt a more flexible attitude to holiday leave, and to move away from the present system of making competing territorial claims.

Case 134

You are interviewing for the post of practice manager. One of the applicants is very suitable and seems to be the first choice. She says, however, that she is a Justice of the Peace and wants to know if she can have time off work for this activity. You are rather anxious about this and feel that it ought not to coincide with her practice duties. What is your response to this request?

It is very important to clarify what the legal situation is. Do employees have a right to time off for this other work? What are the rights of employees? (802)

A knowledge of these rights enables you to respond appropriately to such a request. If you are not sure, you could say that you need to consider this and would let her know. It would be wrong to refuse this request before clarifying what the legal rights of an employee are.

Conclusion

Responsibility for staff in general practice ultimately rests with the doctors and we must ensure that one of our partners has the knowledge and skills needed to be good employers.

Rights of employees include having:

- written terms of employment
- itemised pay statement
- trade union membership if desired
- time off work for
  - trade union activities
  - being a Justice of the Peace or member of a social services, statutory tribunal, Regional District Health Authority, FHSA, health board, governing body of school
- minimum period of notice
- a written statement of reasons for dismissal
- the right not to be unfairly dismissed
- redundancy pay (if fulfilling requirements)
- statutory sick pay
- time off for antenatal care
- the right to return to work after having a child
- statutory maternity pay
- the right not to be discriminated against   [802]

23 Referral decisions

- Uncertainty about diagnosis or management
- Severity of condition or symptoms
- Urgency of condition
- Request by patient or family
- Need for screening, investigations, or treatment that is not otherwise available

The decision to refer a patient is based on many factors including those in the box.

There are wide variations in referral rates which do not correlate with any characteristics of the GP, the patient, or the geographical area. How appropriate are the referral decisions made by GPs? Using implicit criteria of hospital specialists to judge the referrals, Fertig and colleagues found that, except in orthopaedic cases, about 15% were inappropriate, with referrals between hospital specialists faring no differently than those from general practice. Using locally determined clinical guidelines, there was evidence of under-referral.[1] Factors identified by GPs as influencing referral decisions included ease of access, interests and skills of the doctor, patient demands, and fear of litigation.[2]

Other studies have identified an inability to tolerate uncertainty as an important determinant of referral decisions.[3] Uncertainty is, however, rarely discussed in the undergraduate curriculum. The factors that affect the behaviour of individual doctors will also affect referral decisions.[4] It is very important to have clear goals about the reasons for any referral and these must be stated in the referral letter.

Case 135

A woman aged 19 has pain and guarding in the right lower abdomen. Her last period was a week ago. You notice she looks depressed and is tearful. She admits to family stress and problems but will not elaborate. You suspect appendicitis and refer her to hospital. She is told to let you know if she is not admitted. At 3.30 p.m. she returns with a letter from surgeon saying that she suspected appendicitis but the patient refused admission. What do you do?

It is important to identify the fears and anxieties that affect the acceptability of hospital admission   [417]

Before deciding to take a risk, assess all possible outcomes for doctor, patient, relatives, and others who may be involved
                                        [291]

Patients referred as emergencies to be seen by a hospital doctor need to be told to come to surgery or ask for a follow up visit the next day, if not admitted and symptoms persist   [487]

Safeguards may be needed to reduce risk taking to acceptable levels   [292]

Ill patients being managed at home, and their relatives, need information about:

- what to do
- how to identify complications or deterioration
- what to do about them
- when to call the doctor
- what to do if no better within a specified period of time or if condition deteriorates
- when doctor will revisit
                                        [472]

Social factors may affect this patient's behaviour and account for her reluctance to accept admission (417). There are no signs of schizophrenia which may present with depression. She is rational and competent. This patient needs to understand the risks she is taking (291).

Can she be persuaded to tell her partner or family that she is ill? What information does this patient need? (487, 292)

Safeguards that would reduce risk taking include the provision of information about further complications and their management (472).

Follow up plans include a home visit the next day or asking her to come to the surgery. A home visit might give more insight into what the problems are, and there may be an opportunity to talk to the partner or relatives.

Referral for second opinion

All patients have the right to be referred for a second opinion if requested. This may produce conflicting views on management. Sometimes a second opinion is requested because the GP disagrees with the initial consultant's management. It may also be requested to support the GP's management.

Case 136

A child aged nine years was admitted to a local children's hospital for cystoscopy. On the next night the mother telephones to say that she wants a second opinion for her son who is very ill in hospital. After cystoscopy he developed severe abdominal pain and fever. A second operation revealed a perforated bladder. She is very worried and asks you to get a specialist from the teaching hospital to see her son today. What do you do?

> The GP's role includes communication of anxieties of patients and relatives to hospital staff [287]

The mother has good reason to be anxious and her request for a second opinion is understandable. This decision has implications for the hospital staff who are already looking after her son. The first task is to clarify the facts (287).

> Patient or family has the right to a second opinion if requested, preferably after being given all the relevant information about the illness and its management by a consultant [230]

After discussion with the registrar she was given a chance to talk with the consultant later that morning. Afterwards, if she still wished to have a second opinion, this could be arranged (230).

> If a second opinion is requested, this may be organised by the consultant who is already involved and can:
> - select the most appropriate specialist
> - discuss the case with a colleague
> - provide the relevant background information
> - act on any new suggestions without transfer to another hospital or loss of patient confidence [755]

If a second opinion is requested, this can be organised by the GP or the consultant. There are advantages to involving the consultant (755).

After discussing her son's management with the consultant she decided against seeking another opinion.

Case 137

A man aged 54 comes with his wife to see you. He fell off a wall and fractured the fifth and sixth cervical vertebrae. He was given bed rest for six weeks but did not have any traction. He is now in constant pain and has a deformity in spite of collars and analgesics. He is distressed, depressed, angry, and unable to work efficiently. He says he was referred to the Royal National Orthopaedic Hospital where the specialist told him that, if he had been put in traction from the start, he would not be like this now. There is no prospect of surgical treatment. The surgeon said "the only thing that would help would be to refracture the bone and realign it, and no one is going to do that." His wife finds it very difficult to cope with his illness and says that he is a changed man. What is your management?

- To improve function
- To prevent further disability
- To help them to adjust to the disability
- To provide psychological support

The GP and patient must decide whether to accept a consultant's opinion on diagnosis or management, or to seek a second opinion   [202]

A second opinion from a consultant in a different specialty may provide alternative management options, for example, neurosurgeon or rheumatologist versus orthopaedic surgeon, haematologist versus oncologist, psychologist versus psychiatrist, general physician versus terminal care specialist, general surgeon versus plastic surgeon   [560]

The wife and her husband are both depressed and disabled by this accident. The first decision is whether or not to accept this surgeon's assessment. If there is no possibility of further surgery, the management objectives would be those in the box.

The first decision relates to the orthopaedic surgeon's assessment. When a patient is referred to a consultant, it is often for an opinion that may or may not be accepted by the patient or GP (202).

Should this patient be advised to obtain a second opinion and, if so, which specialist should be asked to see him? (560) It may be easier to accept disability when a second opinion confirms that there is no cure or treatment to reduce the disability. Consultants understand why patients make such requests and are rarely offended. Such a referral can be made by the consultant or the GP. This referral was made by the GP but a letter was sent to the original consultant explaining that a second opinion was being sought. He was referred to a neurosurgeon who operated on him with excellent results.

Self referral to the accident and emergency department

Many patients attend the local accident and emergency department. In an analysis of why 217 patients referred themselves, Singh found that the most frequent factors affecting their decision related to perceptions of urgency, need for tests, and availability of their GP.[5]

Most patients attended the accident and emergency department when the surgeries were being held. The availability of appointments was not a factor because patients were seen as emergencies if they felt the problem was urgent. Only 6% had tried to contact their doctor before going to the accident and emergency department. This study showed that the most critical factors influencing patients' decisions were their perceptions of the problem and whether they thought that the GP could deal with it.

The current vogue of provision of GP services in accident and emergency departments is an example of the wrong treatment for an incorrect diagnosis of a behavioural problem. As busy hospital staff do not have the time or the skills needed to educate such patients, it is assumed that patients are ineducable. Meeting inappropriate demands by providing GP services in the accident and emergency department is not the only option. Behavioural psychologists and educators may find other more cost effective solutions to the inappropriate use of scarce resources.

Conclusion

It is important to remember that referral does not mean total transfer of responsibility. It is usually for treatment, assessment, or advice, and the objectives of the referral are not always stated. Never forget that it is the GP who is responsible for follow up and long term care.

1 Fertig A, Roland M, King H, Moore T. Understanding variation in general practitioner rates: are inappropriate referrals important and would guidelines help to reduce rates of referral? *BMJ* 1993;**307**: 1467–70.
2 De Marco P, Cain C, Lockwood T, Roland M. How valuable is feedback of information on hospital referral patterns? Lessons from visits to 92 East Anglian practices. *BMJ* 1993;**307**:1465–6.
3 Newton J, Hayes V, Hutchinson A. Factors influencing general practitioner referral decisions. *Family Practitioner* 1991;**8**:308–13.
4 Hutchinson A. Explaining referral variation. *BMJ* 1993;**307**:1439.
5 Singh S. Self referral to accident and emergency department: patients' perceptions. *BMJ* 1988;**297**:1179–80.

24 Responsibilities

Failure to clarify responsibilities may lead to inappropriate decisions. The GP has to identify the different tasks of other health professionals with whom care is shared. The responsibilities of patients and carers must also be clarified. Failure to do so can lead to decisions that may cause disability and distresss.

Case 138

A mother telephones at 10 p.m. because her baby aged 18 months is miserable and has a fever but no cough, diarrhoea or vomiting, and breathing is normal. You advise paracetamol and fluids and ask her to telephone back in an hour. She telephones back to say baby is now asleep and there are no new symptoms. You ask her whether she would like you to visit or not. She says that this does not seem necessary now. She is instructed to telephone if any new symptoms develop and to bring the child to the surgery in the morning if still febrile. Do you agree with this management?

> Decisions that require professional knowledge and judgement, such as whether or not to visit, should be shared with but not delegated to the patient [363]

> The responsibility for deciding whether or not to visit a patient rests with the doctor [250]

> In assessing the need for a home visit, relevant factors include past and present history of illness, differential diagnosis, severity of symptoms, current medication, recent travel, social circumstances, and anxiety of patient or relatives [583]

The management seems reasonable, but is it fair to delegate the decision about the need for a visit to the mother? (363) Her anxiety about the baby will inevitably conflict with her reluctance to request an unnecessary home visit. She would feel terrible if the child were seriously ill and she decided that a home visit was not needed (250).

The decision about a home visit is one that the doctor should take after assessing all relevant facts. Mothers often telephone for advice if a child is febrile. Should a visit be made? (583)

The child may have recently returned from Africa or had a recent operation or invasive investigation in hospital. There may be a chronic disease such as diabetes or a history of febrile convulsions or sudden infant death syndrome in the family. A careful history is critical when decisions are being made about the need to visit a febrile child. This is especially important when the records are not available.

Relevant information which may not have been obtained on the telephone is often discovered during a visit. If it is decided not to visit, a record must be kept of the telephone consultation and the advice that was given.

Case 139

A girl aged 11 years who was born with multiple handicaps including paralysis, deafness, and poor vision attends a paediatric follow up clinic. The paediatric professor writes to say that, although she is not deficient in growth hormone, she is well below the 3rd percentile and she may benefit from treatment with growth hormone for a year. He asks you to prescribe this at a cost of £5000. You object because he is the doctor who believes that this treatment is indicated and, as he will be monitoring her progress, he ought to prescribe it. He says that monitoring growth is well within the GP's competence. He claims to have had 50 children on growth hormone prescribed by their GPs and there have never been any previous objections or difficulties. The parents have been told that this treatment is indicated and expect you to prescribe it. What is your response?

What evidence is there that this treatment is needed? Her growth hormone levels are normal and there is no evidence of deficiency. The GP must be convinced that good indications exist for prescribing this expensive treatment. The consultant must recognise that responsibility for prescribing is not the only issue.

The parents were told that their child needs this drug. Refusal to prescribe will have a terrible effect on the relationship with this family. Concerns about indications for treatment should be discussed with the consultant. It might be possible to obtain a second consultant's assessment of its need. Such arbitration seems necessary here.

Who should be responsible for monitoring the response to such treatment? It is not clear how this is to be done? If there is no response within a specific period of time, does this mean treatment can be stopped? If response is minimal, for how long should treatment be continued? What is a "good" response? All of these questions need to be answered and clear guidelines are also needed. It is

Responsibility for long term prescribing for a specific chronic disease, for example, AIDS, renal dialysis, etc rests with the doctor who has the major clinical responsibility and this may need clarification   [584]

important to standardise the way in which the response is to be measured. Evaluation of therapy will be impossible if each doctor who sees the patient does something different. If it is decided that the drug is really justified in this patient, then the question of responsibility for prescribing must be discussed (584).

The Department of Health guidelines about responsibility for prescribing need to be discussed with the consultant. The family must not be involved in any disagreement with the consultant. It would have been so much better if the consultant had discussed this treatment option with the GP before mentioning it to the parents (380).

To prevent loss of confidence doctors should not criticise or disagree with each other in front of the patient   [380]

The GP can explain that the management needs to be discussed with the consultant.[1] There should be no suggestion of criticism or disagreement until these issues have been clarified.

This case illustrates the importance of making decisions in the right sequence. The first decision relates to the indications for treatment and its effectiveness in such a patient. If the consultant giving a second opinion decides that the growth hormone is inappropriate then the consultant should explain this to the family. It would be dreadful if they felt that cost was the only consideration and incurred great debts to pay for it themselves. If this treatment were considered the next decision would relate to responsibility for prescribing and monitoring the outcome.

Case 140

A woman aged 26 is 38 weeks' pregnant with her first baby. She attends your antenatal clinic and is found to have a BP of 160/100 and proteinuria. She feels well and has no other abnormal findings. What is your management?

Management decisions about potentially serious problems arising during pregnancy ought to be discussed with hospital staff and midwives who are also involved in shared care   [688]

This is a potentially serious problem and care is being shared between the practice antenatal team and the hospital staff. Should this patient be managed by the GP or should the hospital staff be informed of the problem? (688)

Good shared care involves discussion about problems and their management with relevant professionals. This is

205

Follow up of patients with hypertension in late pregnancy may need to be done on a daily basis and it is important to:

- decide who will visit
- identify follow up observations
- agree on criteria for admission
- educate patient to identify symptoms that need either an emergency visit by GP or immediate admission   [689]

especially important when decisions about responsibility for follow up are made (689).

The management plans should be recorded in the notes so that they are available to other partners. They should also be written down in her shared care booklet. If problems arise, and the visiting doctor does not have the notes, the management plans will be available. This is useful if the practice uses locums or a deputising doctor.

Case 141

A man aged 50 has been treated by a private specialist without first consulting his GP. He was put on oral steroids for what sounded like an unusual postviral arthralgia. This provided symptomatic relief and he felt much better. He returned to the specialist and was given a further month's supply of prednisone 10 mg three times daily. No information had been received about his private treatment and the patient had not mentioned it. He now consults the practice because of thirst and polyuria. His blood sugar is 18, there are no ketones, and he is started on a diet. He has seen the practice nurse and been educated about the diabetes and the diabetic diet, and has been told to return in two weeks' time for a further check. Ten days later you receive a letter from the local hospital saying that he had been admitted in ketoacidosis and that they were surprised that his steroids had not been stopped. A complaint is received from the Family Health Service Authority alleging negligence because no questions were asked about other treatments being taken at the time. What are the relevant factors that need to be considered in your response?

Specialists who accept patients not referred by a GP have a duty to inform the GP of findings and treatment recommendations, unless the patient withholds consent or has no GP, in which case the specialist is responsible for subsequent care until another doctor has agreed to take on this responsibility[2]   [772]

The most important factor relates to responsibility for treatment and any complications that arise from it. The private doctor has not communicated with the GP (772).

This patient was not referred to the private doctor by his own GP and the patient did not mention the steroids. It is difficult to see how the GP can be held responsible for failure to stop the steroids. There was no letter in the records indicating that he was on this treatment, and he had not been given a steroid card to carry with him.

Private doctors have a duty to educate patients about the need to involve their GP and the risks of conflicting treatment or misdiagnosis when they do not do so. Many patients consult private doctors as well as GPs. Perhaps all patients should be asked about medication from other sources when there is a possibility of drug induced disease.

Conclusion

In many chapters throughout this book, problems are presented that relate to failure to identify, accept, or clarify responsibilities. This is especially true for patients with chronic disease, for example, mental illness, who are cared for by different agencies and professionals. The key to good communication and effective care is to clarify responsibilities and ensure that all concerned know what each is able and willing to do.

1 Department of Health guidelines on interface prescribing. EL(91)127(1). London: HMSO.
2 BMA. Shared responsibilities for prescribing. In: *Medical ethics today*, London: BMA, 1993:188.

25 Protocols and policies

Uncertainty

Uncertainty exists because information is often incomplete, the diagnosis is unknown, or knowledge is lacking, and it is not always recognised. It can relate to: diagnosis, knowledge, options available, competence, type of problem, past experience, time available, or lack of goals, policies, or scientific evidence. Doctors need to be trained to identify and resolve uncertainty, and to be able to share doubts with patients. Judgement plays a large part, however, in decisions made by doctors and judgement is fallible. Policies and protocols can help to reduce uncertainty and improve the standard of care.

Disagreements

Disagreements are common among those who share the care of patients. There may be disagreements about the diagnosis or management of individual patients, the organisation of services, or specific management policies. Disagreements may also result from different perceptions of roles and responsibilities. Like illnesses, some disagreements are distressing to doctors and their patients, and can be prevented.

Diagnostic criteria

There is a need for doctors to agree about the diagnostic criteria for certain conditions. Some diagnoses will have profound effects on the social, psychological, and occupational lives of patients. How many psychiatrists in the UK use the same definition of schizophrenia? The failure to standardise diagnostic definitions makes it difficult to evaluate the effectiveness of treatment. Examples of diagnostic criteria include WHO criteria for diabetes, DSM-

III-R diagnostic classification of mental illness, and the Read classification. Failure to use standardised diagnostic criteria could have profound implications for decisions made by doctors, patients, and their families.

Responsibilities

Some decisions are not made because it is not clear who should make them. Is it the responsibility of the practice manager, an individual partner, the accountant? Policies and protocols help to identify responsibilities for decision making within the practice and can prevent disagreements.

Practice agreement

- We get along well enough without one
- We don't need it, we trust each other
- We never quite got around to it, we thought about it but . . .

Some practices do not have a practice agreement. Such an agreement reduces the risk of serious disagreements, and helps to prevent and resolve conflict. The absence of such an agreement may be rationalised as in the box.

When a new partner comes into practice, the absence of a practice agreement can be a decision that all may regret.

- Does the practice agreement indicate how to resolve this issue?
- Does there have to be a consensus?
- Can further information help to resolve the disagreement?
- How do other practices deal with this issue?
- Have all possible options been identified?
- Should a small group within the practice be asked to look at it further and report back to a subsequent practice meeting?
- Could a facilitator help?
- Should the decision be deferred and discussed later on?
- Have all causes of the disagreement been identified?
- Have the advantages and disadvantages of various options been fully explored?
- Have all the outcomes of not making a decision been analysed?
- Would an audit help to clarify the extent of the problem?

- Anticoagulants in elderly people
- Antibiotics in otitis media
- Iron and folate supplements during pregnancy
- Role of diet in treating eczema
- When to start anticonvulsant treatment in childhood epilepsy
- Thrombolysis and the GP

Resolving disagreements

The lack of agreement among the partners may lead to failure to make important decisions. This failure to decide on further action leaves the issue unresolved. What can be done at this point?

The options in the box identify some ways in which disagreements can be resolved.

Decision making procedures

In some practices there is no mechanism for sharing decisions. If this fundamental problem is resolved it is likely that working relationships would improve.

Therapeutic disagreements

When evidence of effectiveness of treatment is inconclusive there is a need to seek a consensus or expert opinion. This can, however, be confusing. The book *Controversies in therapeutics*[1] presents arguments and evidence for and against a particular therapy. A final assessment of the evidence is then presented by the editor. Readers are left to make up their own minds on the basis of the evidence, analysis, and comments of all three people. Issues dealt with include the value of the items in the second box.

Should patients have their gallstones removed? GPs might expect most surgeons to agree about who needs their gallbladders removed. Scott and Black[2] showed the case histories of 252 patients who had undergone cholecystectomy to a panel of doctors of varying specialties and to a panel of surgeons. The mixed panel agreed that the operations were appropriate in 41% of cases and inappropriate in 30%. The surgeons agreed that 52% were appropriate and 2% inappropriate, but could not agree on the remaining 46%. Decisions about the type of surgery pale into insignificance besides the failure to agree on decisions about the need for surgery in the the first place.

Protocols

The lack of protocols means that patients are cared for in different ways by different partners in the practice. This can lead to considerable variation in standards of care. It is important to have a practice protocol for the management of patients with chronic diseases who are being cared for by different doctors in the practice. Protocols are also useful when deciding on the indications for starting or stopping treatment. When management is shared with colleagues working in the community or in hospital, protocols help to clarify roles and responsibilities.

Why do some practices have no protocols? Maybe the need was not recognised or they are seen as a threat to clinical freedom. Guidelines that have been jointly developed help to prevent disagreements about patient management. Trials may not have been done, their design may be poor, or the results inconclusive. When scientific evidence is lacking, guidelines based on the best options available can help to identify the most cost effective treatment. The first box indicates what they need to be.

- Valid and supported if possible by scientific evidence
- Reliable, relevant, applicable, and feasible
- Comprehensive, specific, flexible, and up to date

The guidelines may be international, national, regional, district, or practice specific, and they help to make decisions about the points in the second box.

Protocols help to ensure high quality care and to reduce uncertainty. They are always changing as new evidence becomes available.

- When to investigate and what investigations to do
- What the most appropriate treatment is
- When to start or stop treatment
- Which patients to refer to whom, when to admit
- What to do if treatment fails or complications develop

Type of protocols

Good care depends on identifying what "optimal" management should be. Decisions must be made about which option to go for (see third box).

- Use an existing protocol which represents the "best" current management
- Develop local guidelines
- Adapt existing protocols to local needs

Excellent guidelines already exist for many conditions. Locally developed protocols have been shown to improve quality of care and may increase acceptability and communication among all involved in shared care. Examples of useful protocols for GPs include those below.

International

WHO guidelines on management of mild hypertension[3]

National

Department of Health guidelines clarify issues related to interface prescribing[4]

British Diabetic Association protocols for diabetes[5]

211

British Thoracic Society guidelines on management of asthma[6]

British Hypertension Society guidelines[7]

Regional

Use of radiology services[8]

Royal College

Depression: recognition and management in general practice[9]

Shared care of patients with mental health problems. *Report of a Joint Royal College Working Group*[10]

Local initiatives

Clinical guidelines: Report of local initiative, edited by Haines and Hurwitz[11]

Child abuse and non-accidental injury: Lewisham Social Services guidelines[12]

Clinical and prescribing responsibility at the primary/secondary interface. Report of Lambeth, Southwark, and Lewisham FHSA, 1993

Consensus

Recognition and management of statement depression in general practice[13]

Guidelines for the early management of patients with myocardial infarction[14]

General practice

GPs need to work with hospital colleagues to develop local guidelines for referral and for shared care management of patients with specific problems, for example, for organisation of procedures such as sectioning, and also about how antenatal care should be organised

Such protocols help to achieve high standards of care and provide a sound basis for clinical practice.[15] Excellent and comprehensive guidelines on a very wide range of problems seen in general practice are provided by Khot and Polmear.[16] Protocols are only guidelines, and each doctor is free to decide whether to follow the management suggested. Protocols do much to reduce uncertainty and lead to improved standards of care, teaching, and training.

Breast cancer

Guidelines for managing breast cancer in Britain were published in 1986 after concern about variations in treatment. Chouillet *et al* report on the management of women who had breast cancer diagnosed in the Thames region at the beginning of 1990.[17] Only a quarter of cases had the stage recorded in the notes and only about half the women had axillary surgery to stage the disease, although this is recommended in the guidelines. Management in women of the same age and the same stage of cancer varied considerably, suggesting that surgeons either disagree with the guidelines or choose to ignore them. Should GPs ask their local breast surgeons whether such guidelines are followed or is it none of their business? Would this information affect your place of referral? Is this an issue that the GP representative on the surgical directorate ought to raise? What are the implications for patients when the guidelines on good practice for such patients are ignored?

Policies

- Is a policy needed or not?
- If one exists, does it meet our needs and is it being used?
- What would the advantages and disadvantages of a policy be?
- What options exist?
- What factors affect selection of the most relevant policy?
- What skills, knowledge, resources, or finance might be needed?
- How should it be implemented? By whom, how, where, when?
- What will motivate people to implement it?
- Who will monitor its effectiveness?

Failure to decide on a practice policy can lead to difficulties and unnecessary disagreements. Practice policies are needed on a wide range of issues. These are different from protocols or written procedures for management. A policy clarifies aims and objectives; it prevents patients from playing one doctor off against another. If one practice partner refuses to provide methadone substitution and another does, this can lead to problems when that partner is away unless there is a policy to cover this situation. A policy is a course of action selected from alternatives to guide present and future decisions. Policies are a first step to good management, reducing uncertainty and disagreements, and helping to identify overall standards. The need for practice policies may be recognised by partners, patients, practice staff, or other health workers. When a problem is identified, questions that should be asked include those in the box.

Many cases presented in this book highlight the need for policies about a wide range of problems seen in general practice. Practices need policies for a wide range of tasks. They help to resolve uncertainty and to ensure that the

- Acceptance or removal of patients
- Referral of patients
- Treatment of certain conditions such as drug addiction
- Visit requests when patients have moved out of the area
- Dealing with complaints within the practice
- Interface prescribing
- Structuring practice records
- What to audit
- Repeat prescriptions
- Staff employment, etc

Temporary patients who request tranquillisers, codeine based drugs, or other drugs of addiction are easier to deal with if there is a clear practice policy followed by all partners, trainees, and locums [523]

It may be necessary to obtain urgent information about new or temporary patients from previous GP, other hospitals, or Department of Social Services [594]

organisation of primary care is cost effective and efficient. Many difficult decisions are easier to make if policies have been agreed by all concerned. There is a need for practice policies for the items in the box.

Options have been identified for a wide range of policies needed in general practice.[18] Many tasks are made much easier if there is a practice policy about what should be done. Guidelines can then be developed on how to implement the policy.

Case 142

You are asked by a temporary patient for a prescription for diazepam. She says she is prepared to tail it off slowly but has just run out and is afraid of a withdrawal fit if she stops suddenly. What do you do?

This is a frequent problem and there should be a practice policy for dealing with such requests. When one doctor has refused to prescribe, the patient should not be able to get a prescription from another partner. Unfortunately such patients can be very persistent, persuasive, and intimidating. They often succeed in obtaining a prescription because there is no policy on how to handle these requests (523). How should such a patient be managed? (594)

The patient's previous GP could be asked for information before prescribing. The lists of addicts circulated to practices by the Family Health Service Authority could be checked and the Home Office could be contacted to see if this patient is a registered drug addict. One option is to give enough for that night and try to obtain more information the next day.

A practice policy for management of drug addiction could ensure that such patients sign a "contract" with the partner willing to provide methadone substitution treatment. This would stipulate that other doctors should not be approached for this medication. Some of the problems could be minimised if the special "14 day" prescriptions were used to ensure that only a daily amount is prescribed. Such a policy would reduce the stress that such patients may cause when moving from one partner to another.

Case 143

You are in a busy evening surgery and the receptionist telephones to say that there is a request for a visit to a man who had a tonsillectomy yesterday. His throat is sore. You speak to his wife and suggest that he comes to the surgery. He lives two streets away. She agrees to try and get him down. After surgery you already have another two visits to do, but the receptionist reminds you that this man never arrived. You visit and find he cannot swallow, has a high fever, and the soft palate is swollen and very red. You decide that he needs admission for intravenous antibiotics but the surgical registrar of the hospital where he had his operation says that there are no beds and asks you to use the emergency bed service. You argue that they have a responsibility to take him back as he was only operated on yesterday. He reluctantly agrees to see him in accident and emergency and says that he will try to get hold of the ENT registrar. You admit the patient. How should the issues raised by the case be dealt with?

Does the hospital have an admissions policy and, if so, how are new hospital staff informed about it? GPs were recently advised not to put patients on to the emergency bed service. There was a clear understanding that local patients should always be accepted by the local district hospital where beds would be found for them. Perhaps this policy is no longer feasible. Have the managers been told why it cannot be implemented?

Does the hospital have a policy about the management of postoperative problems? Such patients have always been the responsibility of the hospital that did the initial operation. This may need clarification in view of the difficulty involved in getting this patient readmitted.

Fortunately the receptionist mentioned that this patient had not come down to surgery. If she had not done so, it would have been assumed that he was seen by another partner. At the next staff meeting, she was praised for this initiative. It was decided that staff should inform the duty doctor about any "emergency" patient who was expected in surgery but did not attend. This policy would enable the doctor to telephone or visit such a patient.

This patient was discharged less than 24 hours after a tonsillectomy. Was this the result of pressure for beds or a new policy? The GP representative on the surgical directorate is well placed to obtain the answers to many of these questions.

This case highlights several issues relating to hospital discharge policies, bed shortages, safe surgical practice, responsibility for postoperative complications, the need to educate patients about what to do if postoperative complications develop, and education of managers and junior staff about policies and how to implement them. As a result of this case, the need for a practice policy was identified. A procedure was developed to deal with patients who were asked to come down as emergencies but did not attend.

Antenatal and other rituals

- How many antenatal visits are needed?
- Is it necessary to see the doctor?
- Is it as effective or more effective to see the midwife?
- Is it necessary to record the weight and fundal height?
- Is routine screening of asymptomatic patients for bacteriuria cost effective?
- Is it necessary to listen to the fetal heart as similar information is obtained from asking about fetal movements?
- Is it appropriate to do a vaginal examination as part of the postnatal routine?[19]

- No one thinks that they should be challenged
- No one asks for evidence of effectiveness
- It is more comfortable that way
- The patients like it

Once decisions are made about what "routines" should be done they are rarely challenged. Once established routines become rituals they are rarely reviewed for evidence of effectiveness. Consider the current debate on what ought to be done routinely in antenatal clinics and at the postnatal visit; this may represent a conflict between consumer demand and cost effectiveness. Questions that need to be answered include those in the box.

There are times when rituals persist as a result of the points in the second box.

Sometimes the decisions themselves are taken by others. Steer[20] states that "Current moves to demedicalise and decentralise childbirth and to provide more continuity of care are necessitating radical changes in the organisation of maternity care. They offer an opportunity to discard outdated rituals rather than simply to transfer them from doctors to midwives."

Other rituals recently undertaken by GPs at the instigation of politicians included routine health checks and screening for cardiovascular risk factors. Such policies are inspired by political dogma uncontaminated by evidence of their ineffectiveness and cannot be justified.[21]

Conclusion

Policies and protocols are powerful tools for improving the quality of the care we provide. They help to reduce uncertainty, resolve disagreements, and ensure that care is acceptable and cost effective. If appropriate policies are not developed or if good protocols are ignored, less effective and acceptable ones will be imposed by politicians or managers. The choice is ours.

1 Rubin P (ed.) *Controversies in therapeutics*, London, BMJ publishing group, 1991.
2 Scott EA, Black N. Appropriateness of cholecystectomy. *Ann R Coll Surg Engl* 1992;**74**(suppl):97–101.
3 Summary of 1993 World Health Organization–International Society of Hypertension guidelines for the management of mild hypertension. Subcommittee of WHO/ISH Mild Hypertension Liaison Committee. *BMJ* 1993;**307**:1541–6.
4 Department of Health guidelines on interface prescribing. EL(91)127. London: HMSO.
5 Recommendations for Diabetes Health Promotion Clinics. Published by British Diabetic Association, 10 Queen Anne St, London W1M OBD.
6 Guidelines for the management of asthma: a summary. British Thoracic Society and others. *BMJ* 1993;**306**:776–82.
7 Sever P, Beevers G, Bulpitt C, Lever A, Ramsay L. Reid J, *et al.* Management guidelines in essential hypertension: report of the second working party of the British Hypertension Society. *BMJ* 1993;**306**: 983–7.
8 Making the best of an Imaging Department. Guidelines produced by South East Thames Regional Health Authority, Thrift House, Collington Ave, Bexhill-On-Sea TN39 3NQ.
9 Wright A. *Depression: recognition and management in general practice.* London, Royal College of General Practitioners, 1993.
10 Report of a Joint Royal College Working Group. *Shared care of patients with mental health problems*, Royal College of Psychiatrists and Royal College of General Practitioners. London, Royal College of General Practitioners, 1993. Occasional Paper 60, 1993.
11 Haines A, Hurwitz B (eds). *Clinical guidelines. Report of local initiative*, London, Royal College of General Practitioners, 1992. Occasional Paper 58, 1992.
12 *Child protection procedures*, published by Lewisham Social Services Childcare Co-ordinators Unit, Social Service Secretariat, Laurence House, London SE6 4RU.
13 Paykel ES, Priest RG. Recognition and management of statement depression in general practice: consensus statement. *BMJ* 1992;**305**: 1198–2002.
14 Weston CFM, Penny WJ, Julian DG, on behalf of the British Heart Foundation Working Group. Guidelines for the early management of patients with myocardial infarction. *BMJ* 1994;**308**:767–71.
15 Grol R. Development of guidelines for general practice care. *Br J Gen Prac* 1993;**43**:146–51.
16 Khot A, Polmear A. *Practical general practice: Guidelines for logical management*, Oxford, Butterworth-Heinemann, 1992.
17 Chouillet AM, Bell CMJ, Hiscox JG. Management of breast cancer in Southeast England. *BMJ* 1994;**308**:168–71.

18 Essex BJ. *Systemed*, BMJ publishing group, 1989.
19 Noble T. The routine six week postnatal vaginal examination *BMJ* 1993;**307**:697–8.
20 Steer P. Rituals in antenatal care – do we need them? *BMJ* 1993; **307**:697–8.
21 Burke P. The ethics of screening. In Hart CR, Burk P (eds), *Screening and surveillance in general practice*, Edinburgh, Churchill Livingstone, 1992:35–44.

26 Decisions and the district nurse

Introduction

The roles and responsibilities of the district nurse have changed enormously over the last five years. Their extended role has created new skills and many different kinds of patients can now be cared for at home. To work as a partnership, the district nurse and the GP must recognise each other's special skills.

Case 144

Peter is aged 40 and has had AIDS for four years. District nurses are visiting because he has cytomegalic retinitis and is receiving ganciclovir through a Port-a-Cath. He has a very good relationship with the district nurse. He suddenly deteriorated and was admitted to hospital with subacute intestinal obstruction. Three weeks after admission the district nurse was telephoned by the charge nurse who said that he had deteriorated and wished to see her. In the ward he was found to be drowsy, attached to a diamorphine pump, and receiving dextrose saline through a peripheral line. He was being nursed in a side room with full isolation procedures. He said he felt that he was no longer "in control." He had developed methicillin-resistant staphylococcal infection (MRSA) following a laparotomy for multiple perforations. Since his operation 17 days ago he had received no nutrition and was concerned about his weight loss and increasing weakness. He wants to die at home but felt that his wishes were being ignored. He lives alone but says that he has friends who are prepared to help.

- Patient's wishes
- Options that might give him more control over his treatment
- Willingness of the GP to care for him at home
- Feasibility of home care
- Development of an acceptable home care plan
- Nutritional needs
- Current resources available for home care
- Opinions of hospital medical staff looking after him
- Other options, for example, hospice care, in view of the MRSA infection
- Costs of home care
- Sources of funding
- Whether this is a fund holding practice

Decisions that need to be made by the nurse relate to the items in the box.

After discussion with hospital staff they agreed to the nurse's suggestion of total parenteral nutrition through the Port-a-Cath, and to exchange the continuous diamorphine pump for a patient administered pump to give him more control. The nurse then formulated a home care plan for discussion with the GP. This 24 hour care plan involved district nurses, GPs, the Cross Roads scheme, and agency nurses.

In this case, the patient decided that the nurse was the person who could best act as his advocate. He knew that she would know what was needed and what resources were available in the community. Sharing decisions about the care plan increases the possibility of cooperation by all involved in home care.

Hospital staff often make decisions about terminal care without recognising the skills and resources that are available in the community. They may be unaware of the extended role of the district nurse.

Case 145

Michael is aged 46. He moved into the area with his girlfriend to start a new job. Shortly afterwards, he was diagnosed as having a brain tumour. In spite of surgery and radiotherapy he deteriorated and became terminally ill. Day care was organised at the local hospice. Finally he became very weak and it was decided to admit him to the hospice. The nurses continued to visit. His partner was a teacher and the plan was for him to return home when term ended so that she would be able to continue to look after him. Every time his girlfriend mentioned discharge she was told that it was "too risky for him to be nursed at home."

- Willingness of the GP to provide home care
- Nursing and medical needs of the patient
- Wishes and fears of patient and partner
- Feasibility and acceptability of care plan
- Backup support of hospice
- Probable duration of illness
- Availability of 24 hour nursing cover
- Good communication

The decisions about home care will be affected by the factors in the box.

The nurse and GP decided to do a joint assessment and discuss options with the hospice staff and the patient. A care plan was devised to provide optimum support at home. The patient and carer found this very acceptable. The carer was given the telephone number of the nurse's message pager and the GP's home number at night, and this provided increased security. Doing a joint assessment enabled decisions about community care to be shared with all concerned.

Case 146

Brian is a man aged 34 dying from AIDS and is wheelchair bound as the result of neuropathy. He lives in a charity run hostel, where there are residential carers, but nobody with nursing experience. In spite of pressure relieving mattresses, he has developed pressure sores which are being dressed daily. As his condition deteriorated he developed pressure sores on hips and sacrum which were also dressed daily. Necrotic areas developed over the ears, shoulders, and down the spine. He had expressed a wish not to be transferred to hospital to die, and this was also supported by his mother who visited frequently. The nursing input had become enormous as it required two nurses to turn him and to replace the dressings each time. The nurses working in the team responsible for the hostel realised that they could no longer deal with this workload, and continue to care for their other patients. What options are available?

At this stage it seemed that, in spite of the patient's wishes, he would have to be admitted. This decision should not, however, be made before all possible options have been considered. This patient was fortunate to be in a non-fund holding practice. This enabled nurses from other localities within the patch to help to meet the increased hours needed by this patient.

A fund holding practice would have been allocated a definite number of nurses and it would not be possible to share the workload in this way. A fund holder would have had to negotiate with the provider of the service to obtain extra hours. Guidance from the Department of Health

221

stated that fund holding practices could not buy in services through direct employment or a private agency; fund holders must contract through an established NHS provider. Increased savings could be used to fund the increased level of community nursing needed, but would such a practice be prepared to do so?

Decision sequences

These cases illustrate the need to analyse the sequence in which decisions are made (see box).

The care plan should clarify methods of communication. How often do GPs write in the nursing notes in spite of the fact that there is a page for them to do so?

Case 147

You are working in a six doctor partnership but are not a fund holding practice. Unlike the other practices, you look after most of your terminally ill patients at home, and this includes several patients with AIDS. Two local practices have become fund holders during the past year. The nurse manager comes to see you because she is concerned about changes proposed by the fund holding practices. She is afraid that these practices are negotiating with other providers of district nursing services who may provide a cheaper service. She points out that any movement of a fund holding contract for community services destabilises the organisation that is very small and operating on a tight economic margin. This instability will produce difficulties in providing services to other residents. This would jeopardise the quality of care available to patients of non-fund holding practices. It would also have profound effects on people who have depended on community nursing services to look after them at home, when others cannot do so. What can you do about this?

This is a very serious problem. Decisions made by fund holding practices will affect the quality of care of patients throughout the community. The inability to continue to offer a choice for terminally ill patients who wish to die at home, or to provide nursing care for disabled people at home, raises ethical and social issues as well as financial

- Assess patient's needs (nursing, social, psychological, and economic)
- Assess carer's needs
- Identify what is most acceptable to patient and carers
- Review available resources and skills
- Clarify roles and responsibilities of others
- Identify others who are willing and able to provide care
- Identify care plan options considering:
  —acceptability
  —cost effectiveness
  —feasibility
  —natural history of condition
  —implications for carers, health professionals, social services
  —any existing community or nursing guidelines
- Select option after discussion with relevant health professionals
- Decide how care is to be organised
- Review methods of communication
- Monitor progress
- Evaluate outcomes for patient and family
- Adapt as needs change

ones. It is an example of what happens at a local level when decisions are made without regard for their knock-on effects.

Who is responsible for this situation? It is not fair to blame the fund holders for destabilising the local nursing providers. The real responsibility rests with the politicians who decided that market forces and financial factors should override all other considerations such as equity, quality, and need.

One of the main concerns that nurses have is that GPs will secure the right to employ them directly. If this happens, and the practice decides to change providers, they might lose their jobs. At the moment of writing (January 1994) Virginia Bottomley is on record as saying that direct employment is not on the agenda. Agendas change.

Conclusion

New roles and responsibilities are being developed, and the extended role of the nurse now includes making important decisions with patients about a wide range of problems. Nursing is changing and the ways in which we work together will depend on understanding and working with these changes. Learning with and learning from each other should be the new goal.

27 Waiting lists

Waiting lists seem to have a life of their own. Even those who put the data in are often mystified by what comes out. They are manipulated by politicians, managed by no one, and massaged by managers.

Case 148

A woman aged 80 with severe osteoarthritis of her left hip has been referred to an orthopaedic clinic and is on the waiting list for surgery. She lives alone in a high rise block. Her daughter comes to the surgery to say that her mother is very depressed about the loss of mobility and pain in her hip. She takes no interest in going out and feels like giving up. "What can you suggest doctor?"

> Urgency is assessed by considering the natural history of the condition, the probability of future complications, the severity of present disabilities, and physical, mental, social, and occupational factors [53]

This patient's depression seems to be directly related to her physical disability. It might be more productive to try to alleviate the pain and disability before giving antidepressants. Perhaps the medication could be changed. Could the community physiotherapist help? (53)

> The decision on place of referral should be based on knowledge of hospital waiting lists [263]

Was the waiting list checked before this patient was referred to the specialist? (263)

> Before deciding where to refer a patient for surgery, information is needed about:
> - waiting list for clinic appointment
> - waiting list for actual operation [564]

Knowledge of hospital waiting lists includes the waiting time for an outpatient appointment and for being admitted for surgery. Information about both waiting times should be checked before making such a referral. Figures may not be readily available about the length of time a patient may have to wait for a hip replacement. The hospital consultant or registrar could, however, give some idea of the wait for elective surgery (564).

The GP ought to clarify whether the waiting list has an "urgent" category, and what the urgent criteria are　　　　[226]

It is the GP's responsibility to inform the patient that management options are not only between the NHS and private care, but also between an NHS facility with an unacceptable waiting list and one with an acceptable one　　　　[374]

Hospital staff should be informed of any patient on a waiting list whose condition deteriorates, to see whether admission, investigation, or treatment can be expedited　　　　[736]

Some waiting lists have an urgent category (rule 226). It may be useful to talk to the consultant about criteria for urgent admission. Even if there is no urgent category, the hospital consultant should be informed that she has deteriorated. He may be able to give some idea of how much longer she is likely to wait for surgery. Did the referral letter state that she lived alone in a high rise block? What ought to be done if the wait is unacceptable? (374)

A fund holding GP may not experience these problems, but this patient may find it difficult to change to a fund holding practice. What are the criteria for an extra contractual referral? The case is urgent and the local surgeons are unable to expedite admission for elective surgery. Sometimes the patient's condition deteriorates while waiting for admission (736).

If the patient's condition deteriorates, the GP is responsible for informing the hospital and trying to expedite admission.

Case 149

A man aged 55 has a past history of a malignant polyp removed from the colon three years previously. He has now developed rectal bleeding. There are no abnormalities on abdominal or rectal examination, and he is referred for urgent sigmoidoscopy. The surgeon writes to say that faeces obscured the view so he has put him on the waiting list for sigmoidoscopy after inpatient preparation. Four months later you receive a letter saying that he has just been readmitted and sigmoidoscopy showed an adeno-carcinoma of the rectum. He will be admitted for operation next week. Does the GP need to do anything more at this time?

The fastest route should be chosen to investigate suspected malignancy　　　　[125]

It comes as a shock to realise that this patient had to wait for five months for an urgent investigation (125). Why did it take so long? Are there difficulties getting elective patients admitted for treatment? Does the waiting list have an urgent criterion or is it just "first come first served"?

The GP must ensure that a patient with suspected malignancy, who is put on the waiting list, has been treated or investigated within an acceptable period of time   [16]

Patients with a potentially serious problem who are put on a waiting list for further investigations or treatment should:

• have this entered on their problem list and

• be recalled for follow up within a definite period of time to find out if tests or treatment have been done
                                    [345]

What is considered acceptable and what steps should be taken when delays occur? These are the sorts of questions that need to be answered (16).

What is considered an "acceptable" period in such a patient? How long should a woman with a hard breast lump have to wait for tests to establish the diagnosis? The mental stress on a woman with a breast lump is considered greater than that of a man with suspected malignancy of the bowel. Sex and site do seem to make a difference to perceptions of urgency, acceptability, and psychological distress. Fail safe procedures are needed to prevent such unacceptable delays (345).

The patient should have been told what to do if he was not admitted within a specified period of time. Such a patient could be put on a recall register to ensure that he is not overlooked. The notes should indicate that the patient has been put on the recall register and the records can be reviewed or the patient telephoned for further information after an "acceptable" period of time. If these procedures seem excessive, remember that the GP is held responsible for such delays, and is expected to ensure that such patients obtain urgent treatment.

Case 150

You receive a letter from a hospital consultant about a patient who was referred to the surgical clinic four months previously. It says that sigmoidoscopy revealed a fungating carcinoma of the rectum. He is getting the patient in for surgery within a week. He does comment, however, that the patient is very angry that he had to wait so long for a surgical appointment. You are surprised that the patient was not seen earlier as you had indicated that she had complained of pain and altered bowel function, and this needed further investigation. You feel, however, that the responsibility for such a delay rests with the hospital and not with the GP. How could this delay have been avoided?

The GP may be responsible for a delay in obtaining a hospital appointment or treatment if the referral letter failed to state that the patient's condition was serious, urgent, or had become so while waiting to be seen
                                    [770]

The patient was referred because the differential diagnosis included a growth. Who is responsible for ensuring that the appointment is within an "acceptable" period of time? (770)

> The GP and patient should agree on what is an acceptable waiting time for an appointment, admission, or investigation, and on what to do if this period is exceeded [579]

The letter should have requested an urgent appointment. Not all consultants read the referral letter before appointments are allocated. Such patients should be told to inform their doctor if the appointment is not within an acceptable time period (579).

This period has to be stated in weeks and this advice needs to be written in the notes. A better option might be to ask the receptionist to telephone and make an urgent appointment for the patient. Responsibility for ensuring that an urgent case is seen within an acceptable period of time rests with the GP.

Conclusion

Waiting lists are enigmatic. Little is known about their accuracy or how they work, but they probably reflect some aspects of medical behaviour. Sometimes they are based on a first come first served basis, but this ignores the medical, psychological, and social dimensions of urgency. We need information that is current, accurate, comprehensible, and relevant for the decisions made by GPs and patients. Computerisation seems to have hindered rather than facilitated this goal, and it conceals the fast track wait for fund holding practices. A study of the practical, operational, and ethical aspects of waiting lists is long overdue.

V Specific factors

28 Acceptability

Acceptability may refer to patient preferences or to someone being accepted for a specific form of treatment by a doctor. The first reflects value judgements of the patient, and the second may reflect those of the doctor, especially when specific treatments have to be rationed. The acceptability of treatment to patients often affects the type of care provided and its outcomes.

Case 151

A woman aged 77 consults because of pain in her neck and headaches. A radiograph showed some arthritis, and her haemoglobin and full blood count were normal. She was given ibuprofen. Her son telephoned a week later to say that he is worried about her. She seems unwell and lacks her usual energy. He wonders if there is something seriously wrong or if a tonic would help. On re-examination a hard mass is felt arising out of the pelvis. There is no pain, bleeding, or diarrhoea. She is referred and found to have an ovarian carcinoma. She refuses surgery and wants to be left alone. What is your management at this time?

When relatives' assessment of illness differs from doctor's initial diagnosis, the patient should be reassessed [78]

The doctor's role is to provide information about the risks and benefits, and possible social, psychological, and medical outcomes of alternative options to enable patients to give informed consent [218]

Management may become acceptable if underlying anxieties are identified and resolved [141]

Patients should be reassessed when relatives feel that there is something seriously wrong (78). This patient finds the treatment options unacceptable. Was she given all the information needed to make an informed decision? What does she know about her illness, its natural history, and possible complications? Was she told about the effectiveness and risks of different treatment options? What are her current fears and anxieties? (218, 141)

> Before deciding that treatment for a potentially serious condition is not acceptable, a patient should be advised to share decisions with a partner or family   [416]

> Informed consent is needed for doing nothing, which should be a positive management decision made by the patient after discussion of effectiveness and acceptability of all other available options   [50]

> Management decisions are based on needs and acceptability which change over time   [49]

This patient's son is very concerned about his mother and it may be reasonable to enquire whether she has discussed her decision with him? (416) She has decided that she wants to do nothing. She is competent and has the right to decide to refuse treatment. It is the GP's responsibility to ensure, however, that this is an informed decision (50).

Patients need to know they have the right to change their minds (49). Patients are reassured to hear that some options remain open and that they can change their minds later.

Case 152

A man aged 29 is worried because the hospital doctor has told him not to drive for the next six months. There has been no past history of illness but 10 days ago he was taken to hospital after a car crash. He was said to be twitching on arrival at hospital. A brain scan and EEG were normal. He drives for a living and does not know what caused the car crash. One minute he was driving along and the next thing that he remembered was waking up in hospital. He is very anxious about his job and, as all the tests were normal, he feels that this advice is inappropriate. He asks you what you advise him to do. What is your response?

> Assessment of patient compliance and acceptability should precede selection of appropriate management   [71]

> A patient has the right to a second opinion if advice about fitness for work will seriously interfere with occupation or life, but the initial advice should be heeded until a second opinion has been obtained   [473]

There is a risk that this advice will not be followed (71). GPs often reinforce the advice given by hospital colleagues, but if compliance seems poor, alternative options should be considered (473).

A second opinion will help him to feel that this critical decision has been carefully considered by two independent experts (614).

This patient drives for a living and a further fit would represent a danger to other drivers, passengers, and pedestrians. He was referred to a consultant neurologist who advised him to stop driving for six weeks and, if there were no further problems, he could begin to drive again. This seemed a reasonable compromise and was acceptable to the patient.

> Patients may develop an illness which presents a possible occupational risk to others, and specialist advice may be needed before certifying that the patient is fit for work [614]

Case 153

A man aged 67, previously fit, was admitted for excision of a large vascular cyst on the scalp which was causing discomfort and embarrassment. He returned to surgery very distressed and upset. "I could not go through with it doctor. They asked me to put on this gown. It had no ties except around the neck and all the back was exposed. I couldn't walk down the mixed ward like that. I felt it removed all my dignity. They would not let me wear a pair of the green surgical trousers instead, so I discharged myself." What is your response?

Is this the sort of problem the GP should sort out? (287)

> The GP's role includes communication of anxieties of patients and relatives to hospital staff [287]

Hospital staff and GPs often discuss patients' concerns and anxieties. It is part of our role as doctors working in different places but caring for the same patient. With whom would you discuss this problem? (474)

> To make hospital treatment more acceptable to the patient, the GP may need to communicate with the consultant or ward sister [474]

A letter was sent to the consultant explaining the problem and requesting a spare pair of "greens" for the patient. The consultant was delighted to oblige and said he would ensure that the staff on the ward knew about this.

The patient went back on to the waiting list and was given a photocopy of the consultant's letter to take with him in case the ward staff had not been informed of this promise.

Case 154

A bus driver aged 52, employed by London Transport, is a non-insulin-dependent diabetic diagnosed seven years previously. He was well controlled on diet alone until four months ago when his blood sugar was 15 in spite of good compliance with the diet. He was started on glibenclamide 5 mg daily and his next sugar was 12. The tablets were increased to 10 mg daily and now his sugar is 10. He says that he will lose his job if he has to continue to take this drug. No other job is available. He asks if he can come off this treatment as the job is so very important to him. What do you do?

It is not clear whether the problem relates to his need for tablets rather than diet alone, or whether it is a specific ruling for patients who take glibenclamide. Further clarification is needed. The Transport Medical Officer stated that metformin was acceptable for bus drivers but not glibenclamide. His treatment was changed and good control achieved (281).

> It may be necessary to assess employer's acceptability of patient's treatment before making your management decision [281]

Occasionally the acceptability of a treatment to an employer will affect management decisions.

Case 155

A woman aged 30 is referred to the surgeon because she has a breast lump. She returns very distressed saying that she has a sarcoma and has to have a radical mastectomy. She cannot sleep because of the anxiety and worry about the cosmetic and sexual aspects of such radical surgery. She says her breasts are her best feature and she cannot bear the thought of such an operation. She asks for your help and advice. What is your management?

> Before deciding that treatment for a potentially serious condition is not acceptable, a patient should be advised to share this decision with a partner or family [416]

This patient is very distressed by the proposed operation. She recognises the need for surgery but fears the disfigurement and the psychosexual impact of this procedure (416).

> Surgery for cancer may be more acceptable to patient if GP refers to a surgeon prepared to consider cosmetic reconstruction [406]

It may help to discuss the options with both partners. Before undertaking a joint consultation of this sort, the management objectives must be clarified. These should include identifying and discussing her fears and anxieties. Perhaps other more acceptable options could be considered? (406)

The GP discussed this option with the surgeon who suggested referral to a colleague who did reconstruction after radical mastectomy. This option was more acceptable to this patient.

Case 156

A woman aged 81 has a past history of a mild stroke, hypothyroid disease, and hyperparathyroidism. She now consults because she is losing weight. On examination there are no abnormal findings. Urine, chest radiograph, haemoglobin, and calcium are all normal. A barium meal was done because it was more acceptable than an endoscopy. This showed a large polypoid growth very suspicious of carcinoma of the stomach. The patient feels well and there are no other symptoms apart from the weight loss. She lives alone and is depressed as a result of the recent death of her dog. She is due to go on holiday in a week and is looking forward to this. What is your management?

Would you tell her that the radiographic findings suggest a growth, or would you wait until after her holiday? It is tempting to wait for her to return before mentioning this possibility. The growth might, however, bleed while she is away. She could be told that an ulcer was found. She needs to know what to do if she vomits dark-brown fluid or passes a black motion. Should she be prescribed an H_2-receptor antagonist? Would you give her a letter for a doctor in case medical treatment is needed on holiday?

> Surgical indications and options for suspected or proven malignancy in elderly people should always be discussed with a surgeon before deciding not to refer [467]

On return from holiday she was told that the results showed a possible tumour in the stomach. She was quite adamant that she did not want major surgery. What other options exist? A biopsy will be needed to confirm the diagnosis (467).

Failure to refer for consideration
of palliative surgery when an
elderly person is relatively fit
may result in emergency surgery
in a debilitated patient   [468]

Informed consent is needed for
doing nothing, which should be
a decision made by the patient
after being informed of the
possible outcomes, and the
effectiveness and acceptability of
all other options   [50]

The natural history of the disease must be considered
(468). Doing nothing is an option that needs careful
assessment (50).

The surgeon recommended palliative laser treatment
which was acceptable to the patient. She responded well
to this monthly therapy, and died of a stroke 13 months
later.

Case 157

The senior house officer from the children's hospital telephones you at 10.45 p.m. to say that a baby aged 18
months was brought in with severe respiratory distress.
After being nebulised there was slight improvement. She
felt that the child should be admitted but his mother
refused. She was asked to return to the hospital if the child
became worse. The senior house officer just telephoned
to let you know what has happened. The mother is not
on the telephone. What is your response?

When admission is indicated for
a sick child seen in a hospital
accident and emergency
department, but is not
acceptable to parents, hospital
staff should inform the GP who
should do an immediate home
visit to explore parental fears,
anxieties, and other options
                    [499]

If parents refuse consent for
emergency treatment or for
effective long term treatment to
prevent high risk of serious
complications, consider whether
the child's rights are best
protected by taking the child
into care   [227]

Communication has been good and the senior house
officer has transferred the responsibility for care of this
sick child back to the GP. What should be done at this
time? The family is not on the telephone, and they have
refused the treatment they know the child needs
(499).

It was the father who, without giving a reason, refused
hospital admission. The child was very ill and breath-
less. After 20 minutes he was persuaded to let the family
be taken back to the hospital. They stayed in the ward
until 9 a.m. when the mother took the child home
against medical advice. By that time there was a
definite improvement. What would you have done if
they had not been persuaded to return to hospital?
(227)

When children are suspected to be at risk of neglect or abuse their welfare is paramount, and the social services have a duty to investigate and a Child Protection Conference may recommend application to the court for a Child Assessment Order [836]

If there is uncertainty about consent when treating children or young adults, legal advice should be sought, especially where serious consequences or death could ensue unless treatment is given [873]

This is often a difficult decision and advice should be sought from social services as denial of treatment here constitutes neglect (836, 873).

When parents refuse life saving treatment, the rights of the child take priority over the wishes of the parents.

Case 158

A man aged 50 is found to have a sarcoma of the femur. He says that the surgeon proposes to do a radical new operation which involves removal of the upper leg and top of lower leg, and insertion of a new joint. This operation has only been done on six other people and he is very anxious about the outcome. He wonders what limitations will result and how long it may take to regain mobility. He says that the surgeon has tried to reassure him but he is very frightened. He asks you how long it is likely to take before he is mobile again after this operation. What is your management?

Information from other patients who have experienced the problem, illness, or treatment may relieve anxiety and make some management options more acceptable [384]

This is a difficult question as the operation is new and the GP is unlikely to know about it (384).

It should be possible for him to meet a patient who has had this operation. This would help to answer many of his questions. This option is one that doctors rarely consider. The surgeon was telephoned and was delighted to arrange such a meeting. This made a great difference to the patient. He was reassured to see that mobility was much greater than he had thought possible, and could be achieved within a few weeks of surgery.

Case 159

A woman aged 30 has been investigated for long standing amenorrhoea and is found to have a prolactinoma. Her vision is normal. The endocrinologist would like to start medical therapy but she insists on homoeopathic treatment. She comes to you to say that this is what she wants and requests referral to a homoeopathic doctor. You are very worried about this as the treatment she needs is clearly not homoeopathic. However, all attempts to persuade her otherwise fail. What is your management?

237

When patients insist on homoeopathic treatment, the GP, the patient, and the homoeopath could explore whether it is acceptable to use both approaches at the same time [705]

Patients who insist on homoeopathic treatment may accept conventional treatment if there has been no improvement within a specified period of time [706]

- To identify complications or deterioration at an early stage
- To maintain a good doctor–patient relationship
- To ensure early treatment of complications or problems that might arise

The objective is to maintain a good relationship with the patient, even though she may be making an unwise decision. One option might be to take both types of treatment (705).

If this is not acceptable, she might try the homoeopathic treatment for a limited period of time (706).

Follow up is very important for this patient. The aims of follow up would be those in the box.

A regular follow up appointment is essential and shows the patient that the GP is still interested and concerned.

Case 160

Your practice partner is telephoned at 5.45 p.m. by the daughter of a patient aged 82. She says that her mother has been vomiting and has a painful abdominal swelling. He says that he will visit because she may have a strangulated hernia which needs surgery. The daughter says, however, that her mother is adamant that she does not want a doctor to visit. He explains that this is a potentially dangerous condition, but the daughter reiterates her mother's wishes and says that she is not confused or demented. She lives alone and has not been seen by a doctor since her husband died nine years previously. Your practice partner has recorded what he told the daughter in the notes. You are the duty doctor for the night and he thought that you ought to know about this patient. What are your thoughts about this case?

It is important to identify the fears and anxieties which affect the acceptability of hospital admission [417]

This is a difficult problem. The decision not to visit has been made by your partner and the patient's daughter without reference to her mother. A visit might help to identify fears or misconceptions about hospital treatment (417). Such anxieties can only be identified by direct discussion with the patient. A competent patient has the right to refuse treatment. Perhaps her refusal is based on the assumption that she needs surgery, but she may not have a surgical condition. It might be a medical problem that could be treated at home. Even if she has a strangulated hernia and refuses surgery, she might accept basic nursing care to relieve pain and vomiting. She may decline to see a doctor but may accept a visit by a district nurse who

> Third party information about refusal to see a doctor or to accept treatment must, if possible, be confirmed by direct discussions with the patient
>
> [674]

could diagnose a strangulated hernia and explore her fears. Can you be certain that the daughter is telling you what her mother really said? (674)

Once contact is made, fears and misconceptions can be explored and other options discussed. Patients may say that they will not see the doctor, but when you arrive, they agree to do so. It can be difficult for relatives to make a mental state assessment. She may not be confused or demented, but she could be deluded or paranoid. This would alter the management.

After talking to the patient on the telephone, she agreed to let you visit. The night nurse was asked to join you. She was persuaded to be examined and the diagnosis of a strangulated hernia was confirmed. She had refused to see a doctor because she did not want to be referred to the hospital where her husband had died. When she realised that there were alternatives, she accepted referral for surgery.

Conclusion

Acceptability is affected by many factors including the cultural, social, religious, and family background, as well as the patient's occupation, mental state, and past experience. Its assessment should be made before management selection to ensure that compliance is as good as possible. The acceptability of hospital treatment to the GP is also relevant. GPs act as advocates for their patients, and sometimes the GP is unconvinced of the effectiveness of the proposed treatment. New evidence or information may, however, be available and it is wise to discuss this with the consultant before voicing any doubts to the patient. Acceptability is a fundamental consideration because it affects the behaviour and decisions of the patient, the family, and the GP.

29 Compliance

Compliance is an important determinant of outcome. It affects many decisions made by the GP and must always be considered when the effectiveness of treatment is being assessed.

Assessment of compliance

Before treatment is prescribed an assessment of compliance should be made. Is this patient likely to remember to take the medication? Is there evidence of poor compliance in the past? These observations affect the selection of the most appropriate treatment. Closer follow up is needed if there is a risk of poor compliance, and tests may need to be done to monitor drug levels or responses.

Management selection

When compliance is low, select the management which will be effective and make the least demands on the patient [72]

Assessment of patient compliance and acceptability should precede selection of appropriate management [71]

If compliance is not good, one drug is better than two, and a daily dose is better than more frequent medication. A long acting treatment might be a more effective option. An injection every two weeks may be better than tablets every day (72, 71).

This is an example of a sequence rule, which indicates in what order decisions should be made.

Change of medication

Assess compliance before changing treatment or evaluating outcome or effectiveness [43]

Sometimes a treatment is changed or the quantity of a drug increased because it does not seem to be effective (43).

When a hypertensive patient comes for a blood pressure check, the first question should be "Are you still taking the tablets?" The assumption that treatment may have been stopped makes it easier for patients to admit that they ran out of tablets a few days ago. If this question was not asked, the dose may have been considered inadequate.

This is an important consideration in patients on long term medication for chronic illnesses; this is another "sequence" rule.

Blood tests

In the follow up of some patients with chronic diseases such as hypothyroidism, epilepsy, schizophrenia, and drug addiction, drug levels provide an objective measure of compliance.

Psychological factors

Problems with compliance may relate to difficulties in accepting and coming to terms with the illness and its implications [673]

Compliance may be poor because treatment acceptability was not assessed before selection or because side effects have made it unacceptable. Other psychological factors are also relevant (673).

Difficulties in accepting an illness may occur in newly diagnosed patients with diabetes or epilepsy. This possibility should be considered where compliance is poor. Referral for psychological support to help patients to come to terms with their illness and its effects on their lives might be appropriate.

Risks

Pregnant patients with a drug or alcohol problem may be asked for consent to take regular blood tests to evaluate compliance, treatment, and risk to the fetus [504]

Failure to comply with treatment may affect other people. The fetus may be affected when a pregnant patient with a chronic disease fails to take treatment (504).

When a patient stops prophylactic treatment the GP must:

- identify fears and anxieties that affect acceptability
- identify side effects that might have occurred
- ensure patient understands the need for treatment, and the risks of non-compliance
- educate about how to identify disease for which prophylaxis was given   [699]

Some patients are on prophylactic treatment, for example, antibiotics in splenectomy patients. It is essential that they understand the reasons why such treatment is needed, and are aware of the risks entailed if it is stopped (699).

Patients need to recognise the risks to themselves and others of failure to comply.

Follow up needs

One of the objectives of a follow up appointment might be to assess compliance. How well is the patient tolerating the treatment? Are side effects making compliance difficult? If there is a risk that compliance may be low, further education and encouragement may be necessary.

Communication with hospital

The GP may need to communicate with hospital staff when compliance with medication is poor   [700]

Sometimes a patient is put on long term treatment and is attending the hospital clinic but the GP has observed that compliance is poor (700).

This information has implications for long term treatment and patient education (591).

A differential diagnosis must be made of treatment failure which includes factors related to diagnosis, natural history, presence of complications, patient's behaviour, information given, treatment, dosage, compliance, prevention of recurrence, coexisting diseases and their treatment, and follow up provided   [591]

Without this information hospital staff may change the medication or increase the dose.

Responsibility

Compliance should be assessed before decisions are made about the responsibilities that can be given to a patient. If the patient is forgetful, medication can be provided in a container which contains the morning and evening doses for every day of the week. This can be prepared by relatives or the pharmacist and has been shown to improve compliance. Patients in whom compliance is poor may not be able to identify complications or early relapse. The doctor may have to accept responsibility for these tasks and closer follow up will be needed.

30 Confidentiality

Confidentiality is the cornerstone of the doctor–patient relationship and the foundation for the trust patients have in their doctor. This critical factor must always be considered by GPs and practice staff.

Case 161

A man aged 32 has a urethral discharge following sex with a prostitute. He subsequently had sex with his wife. He refuses to go to a genitourinary clinic but is very worried as his wife is pregnant. He wants you to treat her but she is fit and has no symptoms. Tests showed that he had a gonococcal infection. He is treated but wants his wife treated without being told the real diagnosis. What is your management?

> The doctor must balance the rights of confidentiality against the risks of danger to health of patient or others [203]

> The failure to screen and treat sexually transmitted disease contacts may result in increased morbidity [89]

There is a conflict between the right of the patient to confidentiality and the right of the contact to information and treatment (203). How much of a risk is this condition to his wife and unborn baby? (89)

Confidential information may be disclosed under the following circumstances:

- patient consents to disclosure
- court orders disclosure
- statutory duty, for example, notifiable diseases, drug addiction, abortion, birth, death, accidents at work
- exceptional circumstances where interests of patients are best served by disclosure but impossible or medically undesirable to seek patient's consent
- disclosure in public interest
- serious risk to public health or national security
- sharing information with other health professionals for treatment purposes
- disclosure for medical teaching and bona fide research purposes approved by local ethical committee
- disclosure on a need to know basis to health service management   [776]

A doctor who decides to breach confidentiality must be prepared to explain and justify that decision, whatever the circumstances of the disclosure   [774]

He is very anxious that his wife is treated but refuses to let her be told about his infection. Are there grounds for breaching confidentiality? (776)

Are there grounds for breaching confidentiality in this case? He refused to allow the hospital antenatal clinic to be told about her need for treatment (774).

Before deciding to breach confidentiality it is advisable to discuss the matter with an experienced colleague or to seek advice from a medical defence society or professional association [775]

If the doctor decides that grounds exist to breach confidentiality, the patient should be given an explanation and offered support to deal with the consequences [453]

People in whom one sexually transmitted disease has been identified often have another that is not diagnosed [88]

A woman has the right to know if there is a risk of HIV infection to the fetus, as a decision to have a termination may be based on this information alone [485]

It is always wise to share a difficult decision with a colleague (775, 453).

His wife and unborn child are also your patients. Before his wife can be treated she has to know what the problem is. He needs help to be able to discuss the truth with his wife. He needs to recognise that there are other risks that need to be considered (88).

There is a risk that he has been infected with HIV. Should he be counselled about having an HIV test? What implications does this have for his wife and their baby? (485)

This man had initially decided that the worse outcome would be for his wife to know that he had been with another woman. The doctor's task is to identify other outcomes for him to consider. Would the marriage survive if she found out later that she had HIV or a gonococcal infection? She might respect him for having the courage to tell her and ensure that she received treatment. They could be offered support to improve their relationship. He was asked to think about these issues and a week later he returned to say that he had told his wife, and she was now receiving treatment from another partner in the practice. He said that they would like an appointment to see the practice counsellor.

Case 162

A woman aged 42 comes with a rash on the elbow. She also admits to noticing a breast lump which she is very reluctant to allow you to examine. A hard lump is present but she refuses to be referred for biopsy and treatment. She says that she has just got a new job which she needs to maintain her mortgage repayments. She is afraid that she would lose this job if they knew that she needed an operation. Her husband has been made redundant and there is no possibility of him finding a new job. Even after being told that this may be a growth she refuses to change her mind about going to hospital. She asks you not to discuss this with her husband who is coming in next. What is your management?

If the doctor's "optimal" management is unacceptable, a less effective but more acceptable option may have to be found [145]

Aspiration of a breast lump can be diagnostic and undertaken in the surgery [143]

A domiciliary visit may make certain management options more acceptable to patients [161]

Advice from a consultant may be more acceptable than advice from the GP [167]

Surgery for cancer may be more acceptable to a patient if the GP refers to a surgeon prepared to consider cosmetic reconstruction [406]

Before deciding that treatment for a potentially serious condition is not acceptable, a patient should be advised to share decisions with a partner or family [416]

Could her explanation for not going to hospital conceal other anxieties or fears? Confidentiality has to be maintained but the request not to mention this to her husband says something about their relationship. Optimal management would be urgent referral to the breast clinic (145).

Can the GP investigate this breast lump? (143) It was decided not to try to aspirate this lump at the present time. This patient refuses to go to the clinic, but there are other options (161).

If a domiciliary visit is unacceptable to the patient, would she talk to the surgeon on the telephone? (167) Sometimes fear of a mutilating operation is the main consideration (406, 416).

She was seen on three subsequent occasions and finally agreed to discuss it with her husband, and then accepted referral to the breast clinic. People change their minds and there is often time to reconsider important decisions in general practice.

Case 163

A 22 stone psychotic woman defaults from her long acting antipsychotic injections. She lives with her sons who do not provide much support and they are not on the telephone. She is now very deluded. During evening surgery you get a telephone call from a police station where she has been taken. She is due to appear before the magistrate the next morning. A man who says that he is her solicitor wants to discuss her medical background. What is your response?

The three exceptions to informed consent are:

- emergencies where this cannot be obtained
- where the doctor has clear evidence that full disclosure would lead to severe emotional trauma
- where the patient is judged not to be mentally competent [299]

If the patient's mental state makes it difficult to obtain informed consent to impart information, a relative's consent should be sought [436]

To ensure confidentiality it may be necessary to verify the identity of the person requesting information, and this may be done by telephoning the person back [565]

The patient has the right to request that certain information be excluded or removed from the records, but, before deciding what to do, its accuracy and potential relevance must be discussed [273]

Should this person be given confidential medical information or not? The patient herself is unable to provide informed consent for disclosure of information (299).

Who could be asked to give consent on her behalf? (436) The GP must be sure that this person really is her solicitor (565).

The identity of her solicitor was confirmed by telephoning the police station. Her sons were also present and gave consent for information to be provided.

Case 164

A man aged 35 is very depressed and has personality problems. He has been seeing a psychotherapist but is no better. You suggest a referral to a psychiatrist and he agrees. The specialist recommends drug treatment and writes a three page letter including a long passage about him being gay. He has seen the psychotherapist who has a copy of this report and read it out to him. He was horrified that this was in his notes and medical records. He fears that it could affect job prospects and insurance cover. He asks for this information to be removed. What is your response?

A psychiatric report will always include confidential information and it is rare for a patient to object to this being given to the GP. In this case he had not previously disclosed the fact that he was gay (273). This information may have relevance for the diagnosis of future illnesses. The fact that informed consent is needed before information can be given to a third party does not reassure him. He was angry that consent was not sought for this information to be given to his GP.

Should this information be removed from the psychiatrist's letter? All relevant factors need to be considered and fine judgement is needed. There is rarely one "correct" decision. The information was removed.

Case 165

A man aged 44 has just learned that he is going to develop a slowly progressive hereditary disorder known to impair both intellect and coordination. At present he has no clinical signs of this disease, and psychomotor and IQ tests show no deterioration from his normal levels. He has a very responsible job in which irresponsible behaviour could endanger others. He does not want his employer to know about this illness at present as he cannot afford to retire for a couple of years. At first sign of the disease, he would be willing to stop work and to inform his employer. "Do you think this is acceptable doctor?"

The early signs of this disease may become apparent to others before the patient becomes aware that anything is wrong. Early intellectual impairment may manifest itself by impaired judgement and this could have serious occupational consequences. Ethical issues in this case involve confidentiality, patient's rights, and the rights of others to be supervised by competent people.

What "rights" does the employer have? The patient recognises the possible risk to others, but felt that it was very small at present. He did not believe that it justified breaching confidentiality at this time. Should his employer be told? This man is going to lose his mind and his job, both of which are devastating prospects. It seemed reasonable to offer him a second opinion about the need to inform his employer at this stage. An occupational health specialist, consultant neurologist, or a good psychiatrist could all provide a sound opinion. Everything should be done in a way that seems fair to the patient. He decided to have a second opinion from the neurologist who advised retirement on medical grounds.

This man will need help to plan for the future and to ensure that his family know what is happening. He is not married but lives with a woman he has known for three years. They had hoped to have a family. Both were offered an hour long appointment to come to discuss their feelings and to clarify plans for the future. Genetic counselling may also be relevant and long term support will be needed.

The most important objective at present is to help this patient and his partner come to terms with this illness and its impact on their future lives. Disbelief, anger, and grief are natural bereavement reactions. Loss is what they may now experience, particularly future loss which includes mourning for children whom they may no longer feel able to have. Counselling might help them to recognise and work through these feelings.

Case 166

A GP colleague aged 50 works in a practice with two other partners. She is divorced, lives alone, and has an alcohol problem. She has been referred to a specialist who has admitted her for detoxification three times. Recent liver function tests done by a liver specialist show deterioration and he questions her ability to function effectively if she continues to drink. You call to see her at 11 a.m. because of symptoms of oesophagitis. She smells of alcohol but is sober. She is quite upset at the suggestion that her alcohol problem is out of control and refuses to see the alcohol specialist again. She intends to return to her surgery later in the day. What is your management?

Assessment of risk to patients must precede decisions to allow a sick doctor to continue working [465]

When a doctor is sick and not fit to work but refuses to accept this decision, the "three wise men" procedure may be indicated [459]

There is no doubt that her professional ability will be seriously impaired by her alcoholism (465). This doctor has an uncontrolled alcohol problem which is seriously damaging her health. Patients are at risk as her judgement will be impaired much of the time. How can the GP deal with this issue? (459)

The "three wise men" procedure has been developed to help sick doctors recognise and accept the need for treatment. It helps to preserve confidentiality and can be activated by any colleague and not just the doctor's medical adviser. Each GP should find out what is involved. Advice can be obtained from the BMA or the national counselling service for sick doctors.

Case 167

You are the practice that looks after a newly opened hostel for AIDS patients. There are six patients there, all of whom have AIDS although they are not terminally ill. Your receptionists ask at a staff meeting what this hostel is for. Do you tell them?

Receptionists have access to or are informed about confidential information pertaining to patients on a need to know basis to undertake certain tasks, but they do not have a right to confidential information on the basis of curiosity   [524]

This may seem to be a reasonable request. The hostel is run by volunteers and neighbours may know about it. Staff know about local hostels for patients with learning difficulties and for women seeking refuge. There is, however, a difference between this knowledge and being told which patients have AIDS (524).

The receptionists do not need this information to do their job, and there are no grounds for breaching confidentiality. These patients have the right to expect confidentiality. If the receptionists are told, the GP must be prepared to justify a breach of confidentiality.

Case 168

A man aged 32 comes with a letter from a London Transport Medical Officer. He had been accepted for a job as a bus driver but at the medical examination he was found to have a blood pressure of 175/110. He was turned down on the grounds of hypertension and referred back to you. His blood pressure is now 150/90 on two readings taken at different times. He has a past history of drug addiction from which he has been successfully cured. He also has a drink problem and admits to drinking 35 pints a week. He says that he told the London Transport doctor that he drank 11 pints a week but only at weekends. A year ago he was asked to have a liver function test but refused. He asks you for a letter to state that his blood pressure is now normal as he hopes to be given the job. What is your management at this time?

Confidentiality should not be breached without first trying to obtain informed consent   [672]

His blood pressure is not much of a problem and will not stop him from getting the job. The fact that he has lied about his excessive alcohol intake is worrying as he may be a risk to passengers. Are there grounds for breaching confidentiality in such a case? (672)

The doctor must ensure that the patient understands all possible implications and outcomes of disclosing or concealing information to employers or an insurance company after giving informed consent   [357]

He wants you to inform the London Transport doctor that his blood pressure is now normal. He refuses, however, to let you mention his alcohol intake. Does he really understand the full implications of lying about his alcohol? If he has an accident, his medical records might be requested and consent could not be refused. These would show he had lied and had been counselled about the full implications of concealing this information (357).

In the report about his blood pressure it might be reasonable to enquire whether liver function tests were part of the routine examination. At this time it seemed difficult to justify breaching confidentiality. If there is ever any doubt, however, advice could be sought from colleagues, the BMA, or a medical protection society.

Case 169

The following letter was received

Dear Doctor,
I recently had a vaginal swab taken and on telephoning for the result I heard my name and "vaginal swab" being called out loudly. I imagine a waiting room full of patients in full earshot of what was said and I am not happy about it. In addition, while on the telephone to the receptionist last week I was asked to hold while she dealt with a patient at the desk. While waiting for her to return to me, I was able to hear every detail of the name, address, and personal illness details of the patient to whom she was speaking. I would not want other people to overhear my telephone calls in this way. I feel most concerned about these incidents which represent a serious breakdown in confidentiality in the practice.

What is your response?

> The work of the receptionists must be organised in a way that ensures that confidentiality is not breached when patients ask or answer questions, or when staff give information about results or treatment   [734]

Every practice ought to have a procedure for handling complaints. A reply was sent thanking the patient for drawing this breach of confidentiality to our attention and saying that we would be reviewing our practice procedures. She was told that we would be contacting her again (734).

The practice manager discussed this letter with the reception staff. One of the problems was the siting of the telephone for responding to such enquiries. It was decided that in future responses to such requests should be handled away from the reception area, and care would be taken to ensure that names were not overheard by other patients. The patient was sent a letter informing her of the changes in our working practices, and inviting her to come and talk to the doctor or practice manager about the incident. She thanked us for the letter but did not want to pursue the matter further.

Case 170

Six months previously a man aged 24 came at 6.30 p.m. to the surgery. He was a new patient and says that he has been depressed and anxious for six years but he never told his previous GP. He felt that an evil force had entered his head. He hears voices telling him to drag someone into an alley and knife them, or to throw people under a bus. It took great control not to do these things. He does not take drugs or alcohol. He has been married for two months, but his relationship with his wife is not good. He has three brothers but there is no family history of mental illness. He had never been violent and these delusions and hallucinations have been present for some years. It is only now that he has had the courage to ask for help.

This information is recorded in the referral letter to the psychiatrist and an urgent appointment was requested. The patient telephoned the psychiatrist and seemed agitated, so a domiciliary visit was done. He was started on treatment and was seen once more before he defaulted from follow up. He has not consulted since the first visit.

> Six months later a letter is received from this patient's solicitor. His wife's divorce papers contain a copy of the referral letter. He says that his client is most upset about this and wants to know if a copy was sent to his wife or her solicitor. There has been no request for a copy of this letter. What should be done now?

A confidential document has been obtained by a third party without informed consent. The GP did not provide a copy to anyone except the psychiatrist who recalls receiving the referral letter. Unfortunately he thinks the letter may have been left in the house when he did the visit. There is a risk that this man's delusions may now focus on his GP. The risk is greater if there is a past history of violence. It also relates to the type of delusions experienced (670).

A doctor should be forewarned about the possibility of an encounter with a potentially violent patient [670]

An immediate response to the solicitor should be made to forestall a surgery visit by the patient. If he does make an appointment plans should be made about how to deal with a potentially violent situation. A note should be

> Doctors are responsible for informing colleagues about patients who are potentially violent [655]

> Where basic rights such as confidentiality, consent, etc have been infringed, it is the doctor's responsibility to try to prevent this from happening again [608]

clipped to the front of the record saying that the doctor must be informed if this patient is coming to see you. It is important to discuss this case with your partners (655).

After replying to the solicitor's letter, what further enquiries might be appropriate? (608)

The goal is prevention of recurrence. In this case, it was a simple error and unlikely to recur. There was no intentional breach of confidentiality.

Case 171

A woman writes to complain that a video recording of a consultation she had with you was shown to a group of trainees. One of these included her nephew who had recently joined the local vocational training scheme and he had recognised her. She was asked for permission to record the consultation but writes to express concern at the lack of confidentiality. She asks what your normal procedure is. What is your response?

> In obtaining consent for making a consultation video patients should be told:
> - Why the recording is being made?
> - Who is going to see it?
> - How long the tape will be kept?
> - Who is responsible for maintaining confidentiality?
> - Of their right to:
>   —refuse to have it videoed
>   —have the tape erased if consent is not confirmed after the video has been made [874]

The Royal College of General Practitioners has produced a paper containing guidelines about this issue. Informed consent must be obtained (874).[1]

Consent forms for video recording should:

- record name of patient and accompanying persons
- be easily understood by patient
- name doctor who consulted patient and is responsible for proper use of tape
- state date and place of recording
- record consent before consultation
- explain method of confirming consent afterwards
- record consent of other health professionals or students who were present
- state possibility of withdrawing consent at any time without compromising care
- indicate how tape will be used
- request permission to edit the tape
- state how tape is to be transported and stored if it leaves practice premises
- record time limit for which consent remains valid   [876]

Each consultation video should be:

- accompanied by the consent form with the name and telephone number of the person responsible for it
- transported by recorded delivery
- stored in locked cabinets
     [875]

Consent forms have been designed and can be obtained from the regional adviser's office (876).

There should be a procedure for transporting and storing such material (875).

All the procedures in the rules need to be followed to ensure confidentiality.

Case 172

You have looked after a man aged 58 who has been terminally ill with cancer. He was nursed at home by a long standing close friend. His relationship with his wife ended when she left him for someone else five years previously. After his death, his wife comes to see you. She asks for details of his last illness. She was out of the country at the time, and was upset to learn of his death. During the consultation she requests the identity of the woman who looked after him most of the time. You refuse to disclose this confidential information. She says that she just wants to thank her, and would like her name and address. She then requests access to his records saying that she has a right to this. What is your response?

It is tempting to provide information to a relative of a deceased patient, but the Data Protection Act 1984 indicates circumstances under which access may be denied or modified (788).

One option is to inform the third party of the request, and seek her permission to divulge this information. This is a reasonable compromise.

Access to records may be modified or denied in the following circumstances:

- if it is thought that serious physical or mental harm might occur to patient or another individual who could be identified

- if information about a third party could be disclosed (excluding a health professional who has been involved in care)

- records made before November 1991

- when application for access is made by an individual on behalf of a patient who is incompetent or dead, no information can be given that the patient had considered to be confidential and the holder is not required to explain why any part of the record has been withheld   [788]

Case 173

You are in court giving evidence about a case involving serious domestic violence. Your notes contain very confidential information about the patient's relationship with a third party. You are asked about this by the lawyer for the defence. What do you do?

At what point in the proceedings should confidential information be divulged? (778)

Can a doctor take steps to prevent sensitive information from having to be disclosed? (779)

The court may decide to hear this evidence in camera (780).

If the judge or magistrate orders the doctor to answer the questions the doctor must do so or be held in contempt of court. A knowledge of these basic rules can help to minimise the trauma of revealing sensitive and confidential information in court.

The doctor must wait for a formal court order before disclosing any information in circumstances where the patient refuses consent for the disclosure to be made   [778]

When giving court evidence and before the oath is sworn the doctor should inform the judge if there is reason to believe that part of the evidence should not be disclosed, for example, because it would reveal sensitive information about third parties unconnected with the action   [779]

When giving court evidence, if a doctor is asked for information that would breach confidentiality, the judge should be asked for permission to be excused from answering the question on these grounds   [780]

Conclusion

Confidentiality is a concept that is constantly changing as new legislation reflects the new values of our society. We must ensure that our knowledge and information reflect these changes and are incorporated into our daily practice.

1 Royal College of General Practitioners. Statement on the use of videorecordings of general practice consultations for teaching, learning and assessment; the importance of ethical considerations. London, RCGP, May 1993.
2 BMA. Disclosure. In: *Medical ethics today*, London, BMA, 1993:52–62.

31 Consent

Ethically sound decision making by patients, relatives, and doctors involves:

- a full description of diagnosis and prognosis
- clear communication of doctor's responsibilities, and management options
- identification and assessment of outcomes and complications (risks, benefits) according to their probabilities
- application of appropriate ethical principles to support the management decisions taken   [537]

Rights are so basic and so easily forgotten or ignored. This is particularly true of the right to consent to accept or refuse treatment (537).

In theory, consent should always be obtained for any kind of treatment. In practice there is an implicit understanding that it is implied when treatment is accepted by a patient. Such assumptions are not always justified. Equal understanding of the issues involved is rarely possible. Consent is a process, not an event, and continuing discussion is important.

Case 174

A man aged 70 has bone deposits from carcinoma of the prostate. He has had an orchidectomy and is on hormone treatment. He is active and feels fit. Recently he has developed rectal pain and a tender mass was felt on rectal examination. He was referred and a biopsy revealed an adenocarcinoma of the rectum. The urologist told him that there was an ulcer on the bowel and it was probably best left alone for the time being. He comes to surgery to ask you what you think about this. What is your response?

The doctor's value judgements should not interfere with the patient's right to know what management options exist   [400]

Why has the surgeon not explained the true nature of this "ulcer"? Perhaps he felt that it did not make any difference to the patient to know whether it is malignant or not? The doctor's value judgements should not, however, take precedence over basic rights (400).

257

The patient has the right to be told the truth about the illness unless:

- there is good evidence that harm more severe than temporary depression may result
- the patient has clearly indicated a desire not to be told   [233]

The objectives of surgery include cure, but if not possible, improvement of function and reduction of discomfort, distress, and disability   [379]

In assessing the indications for surgery, the natural history of the condition must be considered   [383]

Failure to refer for consideration of palliative surgery when an elderly person is relatively fit may result in emergency surgery in a debilitated patient   [468]

There are times when it may be appropriate to withold information about the true nature of the illness. Is this such a time? (233)

This patient already knows that he has cancer. He has faced the truth about this illness with courage. He is active and feels well. Without knowing that he has developed another cancer it is difficult to discuss management options. Informed consent is needed for doing nothing, which should be a decision made by the patient after being informed of the possible outcomes, and the effectiveness and acceptability of all other options. Questions that need to be asked include whether it is operable and, if so, is he fit for surgery? What other options are available? (379) What may happen if it is left alone? (383)

He may be planning a holiday and knowing about this new cancer may affect other future plans. What is the risk of obstruction or haemorrhage? (468)

The patient has asked for your opinion. Without all the relevant information it is difficult to discuss management options. He could be told that more information is needed to help him select the most appropriate treatment. This is a good time to explore his anxieties and fears. A useful question to ask is "what worries you most?" It is better to discuss this kind of case with the specialist than to write a letter. It helps to answer some of the questions the patient may have asked, and enables alternative options to be reviewed. The secretary was asked to get the patient's notes out for the surgeon who could then telephone back to discuss this patient. Nothing should be said to undermine the confidence the patient has in the surgeon.

Case 175

A woman aged 37 has just been found to have Huntington's disease. At present she is not disabled and her memory is good. She does not drive and does not have a job. When she was 17 she had an illegitimate baby who was adopted through the social services. She is now married and had one son who was killed in a road traffic accident. What is your management of this patient and her family at this time?

- Counselling to help in adjusting to the implications of this illness
- Planning for future disabilities
- Early identification of deterioration
- Prevention of crises if possible

Children over 16, including those who were adopted, have a right to know about genetic diseases in a parent   [451]

Information about genetic disease can be given to an adopted person without revealing the identity of the parent   [452]

Preconception counselling is important for some patients with chronic diseases or disabilities, or who are at risk of genetic or infective diseases   [634]

Experts such as psychiatrists and lawyers may need to undertake a mental state assessment to decide if someone is competent enough to give informed consent or be responsible for his or her own legal affairs   [113]

The management objectives of this case include those in the box.

Another goal relates to assessment of the impact of a genetic disease on the patient and her family. The adopted baby is also part of her biological family. What rights does this child have? (451, 452) The patient's daughter may be planning to have her own family (634).

Social services might be able to trace her. What if this patient refuses to allow this information to be disclosed to her adopted daughter? If the right of the patient to confidentiality conflicts with the right of the adopted daughter to know of the risk, which takes priority? In this kind of dilemma further advice is needed and may be obtained from the BMA ethical guidelines, or from someone with a special interest and skill in medical ethics. It would be wise to consult the Medical Defence Society.

Case 176

A man aged 24 with learning difficulties lives in a residential home. He has repeatedly requested sterilisation since attending a lecture on birth control. He has sex with his girlfriend who also lives in the same home. She cannot take the pill and he cannot use condoms. He says that neither of them want children and he understands that the operation is irreversible. The family planning doctor agrees to do a vasectomy if he is sure that the patient can give informed consent. There are no close relatives. What do you do?

If there is any doubt about the competence of a patient a second opinion should be sought. In view of the nature of the request it is important to obtain confirmation that this patient is able to give informed consent (113).

In this case the consultant in learning difficulties and a lawyer were both asked to assess his competence to consent to this procedure. They felt that he did understand that the procedure was irreversible and was able to give informed consent. He was subsequently sterilised.

Case 177

A woman aged 50 has a smooth enlarged submandibular gland for four weeks. There are no other abnormalities. Blood tests and chest radiograph were normal. She was referred by your practice partner and is due to see the surgeon in three days to consider a biopsy. She is very worried about this because she fears surgery and thinks the gland is getting smaller. After discussion it was agreed to ask the surgeon to see her now, but to postpone biopsy in view of her anxiety and the fact that it is getting smaller. She was given a letter containing these suggestions to give to the surgeon in the clinic. Ten days later she returns with a scar and a partial seventh nerve palsy. She said that the surgeon was very persuasive but did not warn her of the risk of nerve damage. Another patient had been warned of this risk. Had she known, she says she would not have had the operation. The gland was normal. What is your management at this time?

> To obtain informed consent, information must be given about the risks and benefits of alternative treatments that is accurate, comprehensive, and understandable   [252]

> It is the patient's right to be given information on the risk of surgical complications both short and long term, and how these can be diagnosed or prevented   [411]

What information is needed to enable a patient to give informed consent? (252, 411)

The risk of nerve damage should have been mentioned. Another patient was warned about this possibility before undergoing the same operation by another surgical team. The registrar was telephoned and said that there were two surgical teams on the ward. One always mentioned the risk. His team had no guidelines on what ought to be mentioned and he would discuss this with the consultant. He was glad that it had been brought to their attention. It may be appropriate to inform the patient of this conversation. The GP representative on the surgical directorate could be asked to clarify the outcome of this initiative.

Case 178

A woman aged 92 lives with her daughter and is very frail and has become increasingly demented over the last two years. Recently she has lost weight and become constipated. On rectal examination there is a mass thought to be a carcinoma. The patient tells you she fears and dislikes hospitals. What is your management?

She does not have much physical discomfort except for mild constipation. How does the dementia affect the assessment of acceptability? A patient may be demented, but may retain a clear awareness of what is or is not acceptable. Unfortunately when a patient is demented, explanations will be forgotten and fears remain. When a patient is demented, what was unacceptable yesterday may become acceptable today, and vice versa (298).

Dementia is a serious illness and prevents a patient from giving informed consent (205).

No decision is being made at this time about having an operation. The decision is whether a surgical opinion is needed (467).

The patient and her family would benefit from an expert opinion in which the natural history of the condition and the feasibility of palliative surgery are considered. Failure to refer for consideration of palliative surgery when an elderly person is relatively fit may result in emergency surgery in a debilitated patient. Relatives cannot give informed consent unless they know the diagnosis and what options are available. The GP cannot provide this information and therefore it is appropriate to seek a surgical opinion in such a case.

> A patient's decision may reflect disordered judgement because of the effects of a serious illness on the mental state [298]

> The right of "informed" consent may not apply to patients with severe learning difficulty or dementia, and others may be appointed to make decisions in their best interests [205]

> Surgical indications and options for suspected or proven malignancy in elderly people should always be discussed with a surgeon before deciding not to refer [467]

Case 179

You are looking after a terminally ill man with diabetes, gangrene of the legs, ischaemic heart disease, and depression. He refuses all hospital care and his wife knows that he is dying. She is an ex-nurse and is able to meet most of his needs with help from the district nurses. He has a syringe driver containing diamorphine to contain the pain of the gangrene, and diabetes is well controlled by small doses of glibenclamide. The nurse interrupts your morning surgery to say that she visited and found him sweating and repeating the same words over and over again. Dextrostix shows sugar of less than 1. His wife is told he is having a hypoglycaemic attack. They could not get oral sugar in so the nurse has come down to the health centre to ask you what should be done. What is your response?

- Ask them not to treat the hypoglycaemia?
- Suggest that they give glucagon now?
- Visit after surgery?
- Leave surgery and visit immediately?

The relative has the right to share the decision about whether or not to treat a potentially lethal but curable complication in a patient with a terminal illness who is unconscious

[347]

Doctor and relatives ought to respect requests about terminal illness management when the patient was competent and these may be clarified by advance directives [439]

Rights need to be identified even if patient or relatives decide to waive or delegate them [348]

Good management may include creating opportunities for patient and family to discuss fears and wishes about death and dying

[618]

Which of the options in the box would you take?

This patient is terminally ill. He has been expected to die for many days. There has never been a previous hypoglycaemic attack and this is an unexpected complication, which has presented the nurse with a critical dilemma. It may be reasonable not to treat the hypoglycaemia but who should make this decision? (347)

Has the patient expressed his wishes about care during terminal illness? (439)

In this case there were no advance directives. An immediate visit was done. The notes were reviewed and his wife was asked if he had expressed any wishes about terminal care. She was told that this could be a terminal event if not treated and it could be a peaceful end. She was asked what she felt about not treating the hypoglycaemia and became very upset. She said she did not want to be asked for permission to let him die. "You decide, doctor." (348)

She was not prepared for this potentially treatable and reversible complication. He was treated with intravenous glucose and regained consciousness. A decision now needs to be made about future management of hypoglycaemia or other possible complications. Would you discuss this with the patient or just with his wife? (618)

Such decisions should be recorded in the patient's records and nursing notes. The patient expressed a wish to have no further active treatment other than nursing and symptomatic care. The glibenclamide was stopped.

Case 180

A heterosexual woman aged 34 with AIDS acquired through past drug abuse has a rectal biopsy done in the clinic. Following this she haemorrhaged and had to be admitted and transfused. She has now been discharged. She had no bowel disturbance or pain and was told that the biopsy was done to exclude infection. You telephone the registrar who says that it was done for research purposes. What, if anything, do you do?

262

Informed consent is needed for research procedures and investigations [609]

Where basic rights such as confidentiality, consent, etc have been infringed, it is the doctor's responsibility to try to prevent this from happening again [608]

Discussion between GP and consultant may be the best way to overcome management or ethical problems and meet patients' needs [438]

This patient was not told that the investigation was for research purposes or about the possible risks (609).

Has this research project been approved by the hospital ethical committee? If so, what procedure has been agreed for seeking informed consent? (608)

The hospital ethics committee should ensure that ethical research guidelines are followed. Invasive procedures should not be undertaken without informed consent. Clear guidelines for obtaining consent may exist but are not being followed (438).

This project had been approved by the committee but the investigator was not following the research protocol.

Case 181

You are looking after a gipsy family who live in a caravan encampment near the surgery. They have a child aged four years who has just been found to have a sarcoma. The hospital planned surgery followed by chemotherapy as soon as possible. The consultant discussed this with the parents who seemed in agreement. The registrar telephones to say that there is now a bed and asks you to tell the parents. You last saw the child three days ago when you discussed the hospital plans for treatment with them. You arrive at the encampment to find that the family have gone. They were from Ireland originally. No one knows where they are now. What is your management?

CONSENT

If parents refuse consent for
emergency treatment or for
effective long term treatment to
prevent high risk of serious
complications, consider whether
the child's rights are best
protected by taking the child
into care   [227]

Police assistance may be needed
to find a child in need of urgent
treatment who disappears or
defaults from follow up   [720]

Do you do nothing or ask the police to find them? What
rights does this child have and how may they be protected?
(227, 720)

Would you ask the police for help to find this family or
not? If the parents are found and do not consent to
treatment, would you try to obtain a place of safety order
to ensure that the child is treated? Ethical factors relate to
the rights of the parents and those of the child. The
management decisions in this case should be discussed
with social workers. The family subsequently turned up in
a hospital in Dublin where they had taken the child for
treatment.

Case 182

An Afro-Caribbean mother has brought her daughter aged
nine years to see you. She is worried about a small lump
above the umbilicus, which has been there for two years.
It is not enlarging but at times the girl says it aches. On
examination there is a lump which seems like a small
lipoma. She is a new patient and was seen a few months
ago by a surgeon who said that he would remove it if she
wanted this done. She has now moved into your area and
requests referral to the local hospital for this operation "if
you think it is wise to remove it doctor." What is your
management?

Informed consent for surgery
should include information
about the risk of developing
keloid scars in certain groups of
patients   [690]

What factors affect your decision to refer this child for
surgery? (690)

Obtaining informed consent is usually left to the hospital
staff. It is always wise to discuss the risk of keloid scars
before deciding whether or not to proceed with a minor
operation. After discussion of this risk, the mother decided
not to have this lump removed. Such decisions can always
be reviewed if the clinical condition changes or the lump
enlarges or becomes painful. Consent is a process not an
event.

Case 183

You visit a lady aged 74 who has recently been discharged
after treatment for flare up of osteomyelitis in her leg. She
says that while in hospital a breast lump was found. She

was told that it was a cancer surrounded by fibrous tissue and that it was unlikely to spread or get larger. She was advised that it ought to be left alone. It was not biopsied. She asks you for your opinion on its management. "What do you think doctor?"

It is the competent patient's right to be involved in any decision about investigation, treatment, or place of care [224]

The doctor must continually ask whose decision this is to safeguard the rights of the patient [261]

People may need time to discuss alternatives with others before deciding on the most acceptable management option [326]

Does she want your opinion on management, the natural history of the condition, or the risks and benefits of other options? It is hard to be asked to live with a cancer of the breast. Other people she knows have had surgery and other forms of treatment. She needs to know about the risks and benefits of alternative options. Without this information, informed consent cannot be given (224). This patient has not been involved in a very important management decision (261).

The patient may accept the surgeon's advice but feel that treatment is being withheld. Leaving things alone may be the correct decision, but the alternatives must first be discussed with the patient (326). The patient should know that such alternatives can always be reconsidered. They are based on needs and acceptability which change over time. The patient has the right to discuss management once more with the surgeon before deciding what she would like to have done.

Case 184

A woman aged 54, with a past history of carcinoma of the bronchus successfully operated on three years previously, attends the chest clinic where an enlarged gland was found. On biopsy this was found to be a lymphoma. The chest radiograph was normal and there were no other palpable glands. The surgeon writes to say that he is reluctant to submit her for a scan and possible laparotomy to assess the extent of this disease. He feels that she should be left alone at present as she is so well. He will be seeing her again in six months' time. The patient asks you for your opinion on treatment. What is your response?

To prevent loss of confidence doctors should not criticise or disagree with each other in front of the patient [380]

Does this patient understand what is wrong and what the management options are? This management decision is critical and should be shared with the patient. You may disagree with this surgeon's management and want to

265

Management can be changed without indicating disagreement or disapproval, thereby maintaining the patient's confidence [169]

The GP and patient must decide whether to accept a consultant's opinion on diagnosis or management, or seek a second opinion [202]

When a GP disagrees with a consultant's management, discussion may identify the basis on which decisions were made [381]

change it. Doctors should not, however, criticise each other's management in front of the patient (380, 169).

The patient could be told that, in such cases, it is usual to discuss further management plans with the consultant (202). This decision should not, however, be made before her management is discussed with the surgeon (381).

After discussion it was decided to involve the patient in the decision about referral to the lymphoma clinic. The reasons for referral were discussed and she decided that this was what she wanted to do. She did not, however, want to do anything that would upset the surgeon and was reassured to hear that he also felt a second opinion might be useful. She was referred to the lymphoma clinic and, after further investigations, was started on treatment. Patients respect doctors who change their minds and decide to seek a second opinion.

Case 185

A woman comes to see you about her mother who is in hospital. She is worried because her mother has been put on a life support machine after a cardiac arrest during an operation to repair a strangulated hernia. She has been demented for the last two years but when she was competent she made an advance directive stating that she would not want life support if she became demented and disabled. The doctors have, however, ignored this because she is no longer competent. In effect they are challenging her directives. The relatives are distressed by this and ask if they have the right to do this. What is your response?

What are the grounds for overruling an advance directive? (893)

Advance directives can be challenged in the courts on the grounds that:

• the wording is not precise enough

• it does not cover the proposed treatment

• the patient was not competent to take a decision when the living will was made [893]

Recent court cases in 1992 and 1993 indicate that an anticipatory decision which is clearly established and applicable to the circumstances would be as legally binding as any current decision made by a competent patient.[1] Unfortunately she only registered with the practice six months ago and her old records have not arrived. There is no record of an advance directive being made and her previous GP has died. The fact that life prolonging treatment has been initiated is not grounds for ignoring her wishes. If practicable, treatment should be discontinued in accordance with the directive once it is known.*

The daughter with whom she lives has always made decisions for her during the last three years and she could be regarded as a proxy decision maker. She confirmed her mother's views. This sort of problem is best resolved by direct discussions between the GP and the hospital consultant. It resulted in the life support machine being switched off.

Case 186

A woman aged 73, who is a schizophrenic and has been a diabetic for the last 10 years, now develops a deep ulcer on the foot of an ischaemic leg. She has always believed that people were trying to attack her with knives. She has been told that she needs surgery to improve the blood supply to the leg and to help the ulcer to heal. As a result of her paranoid delusions, however, she refuses consent for any surgical treatment. The leg is in danger of becoming gangrenous. A surgeon is asked to do a domiciliary visit but he is unable to get her to consent to surgery. He wonders if she could be sectioned as her paranoid delusions are preventing her from recognising the seriousness of the situation and from being able to give informed consent. She lives alone. What is your management?

> A mentally ill patient has the right to refuse treatment for a physical illness even when psychotic delusions are specifically related to the decision to refuse such treatment [901]

> The Mental Health Act 1983 is solely for treatment of mental disorder and patients cannot be "sectioned" to facilitate treatment of a physical illness [902]

The surgeon feels that she may need an amputation if she refuses vascular surgery which might improve the blood supply to the leg. It is doubtful whether she could manage alone if she had a leg amputated. Could she be sectioned on the grounds that she is not competent to refuse consent for surgery?[2] (901, 902)

* A BMA guidance on advance directives is also available on request from the BMA's Ethics Division.

- Is this the correct interpretation of the Mental Health Act?
- Could treatment for the schizophrenia improve her delusions and increase the possibility of her consenting to surgery?

In such circumstances it is always wise to obtain a psychiatric opinion. The psychiatrist should be asked the questions in the box.

The patient had been on a variety of treatments for the schizophrenia for many years and the delusions had never gone away. They rarely caused her any problems but now they made it impossible for her to accept surgical treatment. The leg developed dry gangrene. She died two years later of bronchopneumonia.

Case 187

You have a new patient who is a man aged 43 with Down's syndrome. He lives in a local authority hostel and is brought to the surgery for the first time. He needs a repeat prescription of phenytoin. The carer says that he has become unsteady and very withdrawn in the last three months. He has the old notes which contain a letter from a consultant physician, which says that, in view of the recent onset of weakness and fits, he suspects a cerebral tumour. He discussed the need for a scan with the patient's sister who felt it would terrify him. They decided against further investigations. His last fit was three weeks ago and he is now well. What is your management?

The decision not to investigate seems to have been based on the possible fear that a scan might induce. Without investigation there can be no possiblity of treatment. Who should make this decision? What are the rights of such a patient and how can they be safeguarded? These are the questions that must be asked (601).

| The rights of people with learning difficulties should not be overruled by assumptions about acceptability or other value judgements [601] |

| When deciding to investigate or treat a patient with learning difficulties, value judgements should not conflict with ethically sound decisions [600] |

Value judgements about quality of life must not be allowed to affect basic rights (600). Assumptions about acceptability are not relevant to the decision to investigate this patient. Tests can be undertaken in a way that minimises stress and fear. Could this patient give informed consent? He should be given an explanation about why tests are needed, but others would need to consent on his behalf. He is now in local authority care. After discussions with the patient and social workers, he was referred for relevant investigations. These did not cause distress and were normal.

Consent and clinical trials

Some investigators argue that informed consent for entry to clinical trials should be obtained "in the manner considered best for the individual patient."[3] Many studies have shown that patients want more detailed information and that this may help their psychological adjustment to treatment. The case for offering patients more detailed information on the treatment recommended and the reasons why it is being recommended are incontrovertible.[4][5] What is the legal position? The directive of the European Commission implemented in the United Kingdom on 29 November 1993 means that fully informed consent preferably in writing is now the law.[6]

Conclusion

Interactive videos, advance directives, and other techniques (see chapter 71) have been developed to help patients to give informed consent. We must also remember situations where consent is implied but should have been obtained. It is a basic right and must never be overlooked.

1 See remarks of Lord Donaldson, Re T [1992] 4 All ER 649.
2 Eastman N. Mental health law: civil liberties and the principle of reciprocity. *BMJ* 1993;**308**:43–5
3 Tobias J, Souhami R. Fully informed consent can be needlessly cruel. *BMJ* 1993;**307**:1199–2010.
4 Cassileth BR, Zupkis RV, Sutton-Smith K, March V. Information and participation preferences amongst cancer patients. *Ann Intern Med* 1980;**92**:832–6.
5 Kerrigan DD, Thevasagayam RS, Woods TO, *et al.* Who's afraid of informed consent? *BMJ* 1993;**306**:298–300.
6 European Commission. *The rules governing medicinal products in the European community*, Vol 1, Brussels, European Commission, 1989.

32 Culture

All health problems should be seen within a cultural context. Cultural factors affect people's perceptions of symptoms, aetiology of illness, and urgency, severity, and acceptability of treatment. They also affect the responses of the patient and his or her family to illness and its management. The interaction between culture and care is a neglected area of study in most medical schools. It needs to be understood to be able to provide care that is both appropriate and effective.

Case 188

A Nigerian woman aged 24 comes to request an immediate referral for investigation for infertility. She has been married for nine months and has not become pregnant. She is worried about this. There is no past history of serious illness, pelvic infection, terminations, or pregnancies. On examination there are no abnormal findings. What is your response to her request?

> Infertility is a problem that belongs to two people, both of whom need to see the doctor to diagnose the cause [471]

> Cultural factors often determine:
> - the presentation and impact of a problem
> - the responses of patient and relatives
> - requests for and acceptability of investigations or treatment [174]

Infertility lasting for nine months would not normally justify referral for investigation. She could be reassured that there was no reason why she should not conceive and to return if she was not pregnant in nine months' time. Would it be helpful to interview both partners? (471)

Why is she so agitated and worried about not conceiving after such a short time? (174)

The doctor must identify the reasons behind a patient's sense of urgency [175]

Perceptions of aetiology, urgency, and severity have cultural determinants [193]

Initially the doctor did not share the patient's perception of urgency (175). The patient is worried that if she does not become pregnant soon, her husband may divorce her or take another wife. Without this information it would be difficult to understand her anxiety (193).

We live and work with people from many different cultures yet little is known about their cultural backgrounds. Such knowledge provides a better understanding of behaviour and beliefs, as well as differences in compliance and acceptability. It should help us to be more tolerant of what might seem initially to be unreasonable demands or inexplicable behaviour.

Case 189

Muslim parents bring a girl aged four years to surgery. Yesterday she had fallen off her bike. Today her mother has noticed slight vaginal bleeding. Parents are distraught and have cried all day, telephoned other relatives and are convinced that the marriage prospects are ruined as she could no longer be considered a virgin. They insist that the child be examined to see if there was any vaginal injury. The child is very upset and reluctant to be examined. What is your management?

Cultural factors are important in the aetiology and management of stress, anxiety, and mental illness [101]

Unresolved parental anxieties may have long term effects on child development [102]

Reassurance as part of management, may be more effective after examination of the patient [200]

The parental anxiety is very great. The cultural context is one in which the loss of virginity before marriage is a disaster (101). The parents need reassurance that the child's virginity is intact. It is essential to deal effectively with the high level of parental anxiety (102).

Would you examine the child or not? What is the best way to provide reassurance in this case? (200)

Sexual abuse should be included in the differential diagnosis of any child with vaginal bleeding, discharge, or recurrent irritation [711]

Risk of child sexual abuse or non-accidental injury is increased if:

- parent was abused or
- sib was abused or
- sib was on child protection register [568]

The social services have a duty to investigate if there is reasonable suspicion that a child has been or is at risk of abuse, and in making any decisions the social services should give due consideration to the child's religious, linguistic, racial, and cultural background [881]

There is an assumption that the bleeding has been caused by the trauma of falling off the bike. What other possibilities exist? (711)

Sexual abuse occurs in all cultures, social classes, and religious groups (568).

The parents' records should be reviewed to identify any relevant risk factors. Who should examine the child when abuse is suspected (881).

Knowledge of the family, and the past history of its individual members, is critically important. There was nothing in this family's history or background to raise suspicions of abuse.

Private doctors

Patients from different ethnic backgrounds may also be receiving treatment from a private doctor. Some patients may go to a traditional doctor for certain problems, for example, psychosexual difficulties, and attend GPs for illnesses that are perceived to be within their area of expertise. It may be relevant to ask about other therapies that might be taken without showing disapproval.

Attitudes

Our attitudes to patients will affect the outcome of the consultation. Evidence shows that, compared with non-Asian patients, GPs hold less positive attitudes towards Asian patients. They were thought to require longer consultations, be less compliant, and make excessive and inappropriate use of health services. These perceptions have implications for patient care, workload, and teaching.[1]

Obstetric care

Many Asian women are unable to accept antenatal care provided by a male doctor. This may account for a low attendance in some ethnic groups. The higher perinatal mortality in this group of women may reflect a combination of higher risk and use of an unacceptable antenatal service.

The training of midwives from our indigenous Asian communities could do much to improve the uptake and acceptability of antenatal care.

Prevention

Asian women have a much greater risk of developing osteomalacia and this knowledge should highlight the need for prevention. Does the hospital have a policy for the prevention of this condition in high risk Asian women? If so, how can this be achieved? The GP representative on the obstetric and gynaecology directorates should discuss this with the hospital staff. Are vitamin D and calcium given routinely to high risk groups? What training do junior staff have in the prevention of this disease? There have been countless Royal Commissions on this issue yet little impact has been made on daily preventive practice.

Diabetics

All new Asian diabetic individuals should be referred to a dietician who understands the diets of Asian patients and preferably who speaks their language or has literature in relevant languages. How often is this done?

Conclusion

The study of culture in a medical context is gaining in popularity.[2] Courses in medical anthropology offer doctors insight into the way culture and sociology affect behaviours related to sickness and health. More needs to be done at undergraduate and postgraduate level to improve our understanding of this neglected field which has much to contribute to general practice.

1 Ahmad WI, Baker MR, Kernohan EE. General Practitioners' perceptions of Asian and non-Asian patients. *Fam Pract* 1991;**8**(1):52–6.
2 Qureshi, B. *Dealing with patients from other cultures*, 2nd edn, London, Kluwer Academic Press, 1994.

33 Risk

If you want to practise prevention, think risk. Risk factors are relevant in many decisions made about diagnosis, management, and follow up. The concept of risk needs to be introduced early in the undergraduate curriculum, and it must relate to problems encountered in general practice.

Case 190

A patient aged 17 is 12 weeks' pregnant and lives with her boyfriend in a squatters' community. She has no contact with her family who live 400 miles away. She is known to have been treated for heroin addiction six months previously, but failed to complete the treatment. She is anxious about the baby, insists on a home delivery, and is reluctant to attend the antenatal clinic. She has defaulted on the first two appointments. She is not considered suitable for a home delivery which is an option offered by the practice. What is your management?

How should risk be assessed in early pregnancy? (505)

Assessment of risk in pregnancy includes history of:

- mental illness
- child taken into care
- child on child protection register
- patient or partner at high risk for HIV or hepatitis
- alcohol or drug problems
- housing problems
- single parents living alone
- ethnic minorities at risk of osteomalacia
- medical and obstetric risk factors   [505]

Babies are at risk of passively acquiring the diseases that may complicate drug addiction, for example, HIV and hepatitis B infection [316]

A woman has the right to know if there is a risk of HIV infection to the fetus, because a decision to have a termination may be based on this information alone [485]

For effective management of chronic disease, alcohol problems, and addiction, care needs to be shared and, to do this, the responsibility and tasks of each person, including the patient, should be clearly identified and acceptable to all concerned [286]

Antenatal defaulters have a higher morbidity and perinatal mortality, and need careful follow up [133]

High risk pregnant women who do not attend antenatal clinic may need follow up antenatal care at home [714]

Home delivery for high risk women may be the only acceptable option if the patient accepts the risks, because the alternative may be no care at all [234]

There is a risk that this baby could develop infections transmitted by the mother (316). The mother's anxiety is understandable and further information is needed to assess the risk. Would she want this baby if there were a high risk of HIV infection? (485)

A test for hepatitis B is part of the antenatal screening. If she is a carrier, decisions about immunising the baby will have to be made later. It is important to identify any current behaviours that place her at risk of HIV infection. Do they use a needle exchange system? Her anxiety about attending hospital must be explored. Many such patients fear that infection control procedures will identify them to other mothers as HIV carriers.

This patient's care is shared among the members of the team looking after her pregnancy, and the team dealing with her drug addiction. Each must know what the goals and management plans are (286).

This patient has defaulted from antenatal care in the health centre and is a high risk patient (133). A decision must be made about the provision of domiciliary antenatal care (714).

The home circumstances are poor, but doctors and midwives sometimes have to provide care in suboptimal conditions (234).

> For some high risk patients shared care in pregnancy may mean formulating management plans by discussion with patient, GP, obstetrician, and a specialist in alcohol or drug addiction
> [508]

> Pregnant patients with a drug or alcohol problem may be asked for consent to take regular blood tests to evaluate compliance, treatment, and risk to the fetus [504]

> Urgent discussions with the Department of Social Services or an interagency meeting may be needed to assess the risk to the unborn child and, if there is sufficient concern, a pre-birth child protection case conference may be considered [880]

This mother and baby have special needs. Management should be shared with relevant staff and much of her care may have to be provided at home (508).

Hospital care is not acceptable at this time, but complications might arise which could make this a life saving option. If possible, written informed consent should be obtained for admission to hospital under such circumstances. The obstetrician and paediatrician need to know about this case. They can still share decisions about care and advise on current management even if they have not seen the patient. The drug addiction will need careful supervision (504).

There is a high risk to the baby immediately after birth. If the mother continues to take heroin throughout her pregnancy there is high risk to the baby who may need hospital admission after birth. What should be done if she has been taking heroin before the birth, but refuses to allow the baby to be admitted? Are there grounds for having the baby taken into care? The Children Act provides guidelines for such situations (880).

The GP must alert other relevant agencies to the potential risks that face some unborn children. Good communication about progress, complications, relapses, and defaulting from antenatal care is essential to try to ensure effective care. There should be shared goals and plans for monitoring care before, during, and after birth. The GP must liaise with the addiction specialist, paediatrician, midwife, obstetrician, and social worker, as well as the patient.

An agreed plan should be drawn up and sent to all relevant professionals. The patient should also be given one. This clarifies responsibilities and forms a "contract" between the patient and others involved in her care. What is unacceptable in early pregnancy may well become acceptable later on.

Case 191

An elegant Afro-Caribbean woman aged 44 requests a private referral for cosmetic breast surgery. She feels that her breasts sag and are ugly. "They used to be my best feature, doctor." Her husband has reassured her that he still finds her very attractive and sex is good. However, she cannot bear to look at herself naked and does not accept his reassurances. It constantly plays on her mind and is becoming her sole preoccupation, causing her to feel depressed and sad. There are no other features of depressive illness. She really would like to be referred. What is your management?

Assessment of patient's mental state should precede decision to refer for cosmetic surgery [323]

It is in the patient's own interest to allow GP to select referral consultant rather than relying on self selection [458]

Before counselling someone on the advisability of surgery, the risks and benefits must be assessed [58]

Afro-Caribbeans and Africans have a higher risk of developing keloid scars than other patients and it may be relevant to inform them of this surgical complication [325]

Is her mental state a result of her body image or could her low self image be the presentation of a depressive illness? (323)

There were no features suggestive of a primary depressive illness. It seemed reasonable to agree to this referral. If it is refused, she might select a surgeon herself, whose competence is unknown (458, 58, 325).

She was referred privately to a plastic surgeon known to be conservative and only operating when there were clear indications. He felt that there was a very high risk of keloid scars which could make her appearance much worse and that she would be better off without surgery. She was able to accept his advice.

This patient needs a follow up assessment. Has her mood changed for the better? Has she come to terms with her appearance? Is she still depressed and unhappy? Does she need antidepressant treatment, counselling, or psychological referral? At follow up she was well, and felt much better about herself.

Case 192

A man aged 25 is a new patient who has recently been in prison. He has no past history of serious illness and his only complaint is of weight loss. Urine, chest radiograph, full blood count, and erythrocyte sedimentation rate were all normal. You wonder about AIDS, and he admits to being bisexual and using intravenous heroin until 14 months ago. He lives with a woman aged 20 years. They have a child aged two years, and she is now pregnant with twins. You mention the possibility of AIDS and he admits to suspecting this or cancer. "If I knew I had AIDS I would top myself, doctor." What is your management?

Counselling for the HIV test should be postponed in anyone with a mental illness or disturbed mental state until this has been treated [640]

A drug addict may spread infection, for example, hepatitis and HIV, to others at risk who may need to be screened or immunised [691]

High risk of HIV infection is accompanied by high risk of being a hepatitis B carrier and, if informed consent is given for the HIV test, the patient usually also agrees to hepatitis B test [528]

If mother or partner has a history of intravenous drug abuse, consent should be obtained to record HIV risk on the problem lists of children and spouse [531]

It takes time to come to terms with this possibility. The patient may not understand the natural history of the disease, or may feel that there is no treatment for any of its complications. Time is needed for a longer consultation where fears can be explored and the patient can learn about the illness and its treatment (640).

Most districts have HIV counsellors and the GP must decide whether the patient should be counselled in the surgery or referred to an HIV counsellor (691).

Does his partner have the right to know about the HIV risks to herself and the children? What other risks might this family have been exposed to? (528)

Both partners should be screened for hepatitis B. If he is a hepatitis B carrier and she is not, subsequent plans should include immunisation for her and the babies.

Do the obstetric team know the social background of this couple? Management of this pregnancy and labour should be undertaken as if she were HIV positive. Her notes should be examined to see if the risks have been declared. If not, the importance of informing the hospital staff about the HIV risk should be discussed.

Knowledge about the HIV risk is relevant to any doctor caring for anyone in this family. How can other practice partners be made aware of this risk? Is consent needed to record this information on their problem lists? What implications will this have for patient confidentiality? (531)

Case 193

An Asian woman aged 30 is pregnant. She has three children and lives in poor social and domestic circumstances. She has arranged for a private termination and you sign the form as requested. You mention that she has been a hepatitis B carrier since her hepatitis four years ago. A week later she returns to say that they refused to do the termination because of her hepatitis tests. She is now 12 weeks' pregnant and the local hospital refuses to do patients after 12 weeks. Pregnancy Advisory Service and Brook St Advisory Centre and two local gynaecologists all refuse because of her hepatitis carrier status. What is your management now?

<table>
<tr><td>

Referral of hepatitis B carriers for termination of pregnancy or other surgical procedures is best made to a hospital used to dealing with such patients, for example, HIV positive patients needing surgery [586]

</td></tr>
</table>

It was a surprise to discover how many hospitals and clinics refused to help this patient. The same reluctance is found, however, in obtaining surgery for HIV positive patients (586).

The best option is to find a hospital that provides surgery for this group of patients. This is appropriate because many HIV positive patients are also hepatitis B carriers. After discussion with the gynaecology registrar at the hospital that dealt with most of the HIV positive patients, she was accepted for a termination of pregnancy. As the practice is not fund holding and there was no contract for purchasing services from this hospital, an urgent extra contractual request was made for this referral. What other relevant objectives should be considered in this case? (107)

<table>
<tr><td>

An important management objective is to prevent problems in the adult, child, and fetus at risk [107]

</td></tr>
</table>

<table>
<tr><td>

Patients, relatives and contacts at high risk of being a hepatitis B carrier should be asked for consent to be screened for this condition [527]

</td></tr>
</table>

<table>
<tr><td>

To prevent hepatitis, GPs should use DoH guidelines to identify high risk behaviours, occupations, and groups who need to be screened and possibly immunised [529]

</td></tr>
</table>

Have relatives been screened for hepatitis B? (527) If the husband is negative he ought to be immunised. Was the baby immunised at birth? The records indicate that the paediatrician thought that this was not necessary. The child is now 18 months old (529). The paediatrician's opinion should be considered alongside current Department of Health guidelines. Had these been followed, the baby would have been immunised at birth. The husband was screened and found to be negative. The father and children were immunised against hepatitis B.

Case 194

A woman aged 41 smokes 15 cigarettes a day and does not want to stop smoking. She wants to continue taking the Pill and refuses all alternative forms of contraception. She says that she accepts the risks this entails. Do you prescribe the Pill for her or not?

<table>
<tr><td>

Information given to patients about specific risks of treatment should be clearly recorded in the notes [617]

</td></tr>
</table>

The patient was told of the risks and is willing to accept them. If a serious complication develops there should be some evidence that the risks were discussed (617).

Patient may request a specific treatment and be willing to accept its risks, but doctor may refuse to provide it if its risks are higher than other equally effective available options   [604]

A patient who requests a specific or a new treatment needs information about its risks, benefits, and cost effectiveness, as well as alternative options so that an informed decision can be made   [418]

Patients have the right to take a risk but this may conflict with the doctor's right to refuse to prescribe (604).

Patients have to be allowed to make decisions that doctors may disagree with (418).

Provided risks are clearly presented, understood, and documented, it may be appropriate to agree to her request to continue the Pill. A strong case can be made for disagreeing with this conclusion.

Case 195

A woman aged 22 comes for a repeat prescription for the Pill. She is also worried about the man aged 30 she has been living with for the last 18 months. He is not your patient. Recently he has become very withdrawn and says his GP has diagnosed glandular fever as a cause of his malaise and enlarged glands. He used to be a drug addict but was cured two years ago and there have been no relapses. She asks you if glandular fever is very infectious and how long it takes to get better. What is your response?

A partner or contact has a right to know about risk of exposure to an infectious disease   [606]

A patient, partner, or relative may present with a problem that relates to someone registered with another GP, and effective communication with others, which safeguards confidentiality, may be needed to resolve the problem   [329]

This is your patient and she has a right to know whether her partner has AIDS (606).

Would you contact the GP who is looking after her partner? (329)

Some problems cannot be managed effectively until the truth has been accepted by patient and partner, and this may be done best by a home visit [612]

The right to confidentiality means that consent is needed before a GP can discuss a patient's problem with relatives or others, for example, another GP [330]

The objectives of the consultation are to:
- identify and manage acute illness
- review management of coexisting chronic illness
- screen for health problems and risk factors, and prevent or treat as necessary
- modify future help seeking behaviour where appropriate [375]

An important management objective is to prevent osteomalacia and infectious diseases in high risk groups of adults and children [108]

Patients, relatives, and contacts at high risk of being a hepatitis B carrier should be asked for consent to be screened for this condition [527]

Your colleague may not know about the past history of drug abuse, and may not have considered AIDS. If this is the real diagnosis, joint discussion may identify the most appropriate way to help them both (612, 330).

Even if your colleague declines to give you any information, he or she will now be aware of the special needs and anxieties of your patient.

Case 196

A Vietnamese man aged 38 comes as a new patient. He is married and has three children below the age of nine years. His old notes indicate no serious past illnesses or allergies. He has otitis media which you treat. His blood pressure is normal, and he is a non-smoker. What other considerations are relevant?

The management of this patient will depend on the doctor's perception of the goals of the consultation (375).

What are the relevant risk factors in this case? (108)

This patient is Vietnamese and there is a high risk of him being a hepatitis B carrier. Another appointment was organised, and an interpreter was arranged (527).

He was found to be hepatitis B positive and his wife and children are also at risk. The interpreter explained why the family needed to be screened and why immunisation might be advisable. His family were all hepatitis B negative and were subsequently immunised. What would you have done if the children were carriers?

Case 197

A woman comes to see you on a Thursday evening to discuss what immunisations she should have to go to Uganda. She tells you that she is 12 weeks' pregnant. She is a management consultant working for the World Bank. She has been looking forward to this very important assignment and she will be there for six weeks. What is your management?

> Patients who intend to travel to
> a developing country in early
> pregnancy need to know that
> there is a 20% risk of
> miscarriage and a high risk of
> HIV infection should a blood
> transfusion be necessary   [732]

This patient is excited about going to Africa and the objective of such a consultation would be to prevent infectious diseases by appropriate immunisation and anti-malarial treatment. What else needs to be considered? (732)

Any miscarriage may necessitate a blood transfusion, and in a developing country there would be a high risk of HIV infection. At this point she became very upset. She only came for travel advice but now she must choose between her desire to go and her need to avoid unnecessary risks to herself and the fetus. It was suggested that she might like to have some time to think things over and discuss the possibilities with her partner. She was offered a longer appointment the following week.

When she returned she had decided not to go to Africa. She said that her boss was very understanding. It was a disappointment but she was very happy about the pregnancy and felt that she had made the right decision. Would this issue have been raised if she had gone to the nurse run travel clinic? This problem was discussed with the nurses and it was agreed to refer all such cases to the GP before providing the necessary immunisation advice.

Case 198

A married couple come to see you because they want a child. The wife is aged 32 and this is her first marriage. She has been investigated for infertility, and GIFT (gamete in vitro fertilisation technique) has failed to help her conceive. Her husband is 38 and this is his second marriage. He has had a child by his first wife. They say that they have found someone who would be willing to act as a surrogate and who totally understands their predicament. This is a friend who has had a child of her own and who really wants to help them. She also happens to be a patient of yours. They have only come to inform you about this, and to let you know the background before the surrogate mother attends your antenatal clinic. What is your response?

When surrogate pregnancy is requested it is important to:

- give first priority to welfare of the potential child

- consider this option only when all other means of conception have been tried and failed

- only consider women as potential surrogates who have partners and have already had one or more children

- ensure the commissioning couple and the surrogate mother do not know each other's identity [811]

Risks of genetic disease should be identified to prospective parents before conception [160]

The Surrogacy Arrangements Act 1985 prohibits commercial surrogacy arrangements but permits non-commercial activities and does not ban payment of expenses to a surrogate mother. It is encouraging that this couple have confided their plans to the GP. The 1990 British Medical Association report contains brief guidelines for doctors (811, 160).[1]

These rules form the basis for counselling this couple. This is a specialist field, however, and it may be advisable to refer them to someone who is familiar with issues surrounding surrogate pregnancies.

Case 199

A woman aged 23 requests a home visit. She is 10 weeks' pregnant and complains of severe headaches for the last two months. For the last five days the headaches have been accompanied by vomiting in the mornings. She also complains of feeling weak and drowsy at times. There are no abnormal findings on clinical examination. She is referred for an urgent neurological assessment and has a brain scan and a lumbar puncture, both of which are normal. Four weeks later she comes to the surgery as an emergency with her husband and her 14 month old son. They are very agitated because they have found out the cause of the headaches. There was a blocked flue in their house which has caused high levels of carbon monoxide to build up. This was discovered yesterday by the gas people who were called in because they smelt gas. She is now 14 weeks' pregnant and is very worried by the effect this may have had on the fetus. Since repairing the flue her headaches have gone and she feels much better. You do a carboxyhaemoglobin level which is negative. She wants reassurance that the baby will not have been harmed. "If there was any chance that the baby would have been affected, I would want a termination." What is your management?

- Reassure her that the risk would be very small

- Do a scan and, if normal, reassure her

- Take further advice

She now feels much better and there is no carboxyhaemoglobin in the blood. How do you assess the risk to the fetus? You could do any of the options in the box.

Management will depend on the probability of risk to the

fetus. Although this may be considered to be low, would you obtain further advice and, if so, from whom? Initially she was reassured that it would be most unlikely to have caused any damage to the fetus. However, after the couple had left, a nagging doubt was felt because this critical management decision was made on the basis of an impression and not on factual information. The poisons unit was phoned to confirm the GP's impression.

The risk was much higher than the GP had thought. In view of the length of exposure and the stage of pregnancy, there could be a 20% probability of neurological developmental abnormality. As a result of this information the clinical toxicology specialist was telephoned and agreed to see the couple the following day. They were asked to reattend surgery that evening when they were told of the information from the poisons unit. Because the risk was not as small as initially thought, it seemed advisable to discuss this with the toxicology specialist. They finally decided to have the pregnancy terminated. Follow up support and perhaps counselling are always needed after a termination for whatever reason.

Doctors who may be a risk to patients

Doctors are sometimes a risk to their patients. This may be because of the following factors:

- Physical or mental illness
- Lack of knowledge or competence
- Poor decision making skills

All of us present risks to patients because judgement is always fallible. The risks to patients can, however, be reduced under the following circumstances.

- When there is time to listen and take a careful history
- When information is:
  —comprehensive
  —structured
  —retrievable
- When management is based on evidence of effectiveness
- When all relevant factors are considered
- When all relevant decisions are identified
- When decisions are made in the right sequence

- When patients are educated about their illness, treatment, and responsibilities
- When patients share in the decision making process
- When goals are clearly identified by doctor and patient
- When there is good communication between GP and others involved in care in a hospital or the community
- When care is organised in a cost effective, safe, and acceptable manner
- When doctors are prepared to admit and learn from mistakes
- When limits are recognised and efforts made to reduce uncertainty

We need to test the hypothesis that doctors educated in decision making skills present less of a risk to patients.

Children at risk of serious illness

The identification of babies under six months of age who have serious illness is of great importance. What are the best predictors of serious illness and how can this information be used to educate parents and doctors? Morley et al[2] developed a scoring system to grade the severity of acute systemic illness in babies under six months of age. Data were collected on 28 symptoms and 47 signs from 1007 babies with a spectrum of illness ranging from mild to serious. Regression analysis identified 19 symptoms and signs which most accurately predicted the severity of illness. These were then converted into an accurate scoring system for use by parents and professionals.[3] The Baby Check scoring system is a highly sensitive and specific tool to help decide how severely ill a baby really is. It is not a substitute for common sense or experience, but is a decision aid to help quantify the severity of an illness. The scores can be done at different times to assess improvement or deterioration.

> Examples of Baby Check can be obtained from Baby Check, PO Box 324, Wroxham, Norwich NR12 8EQ.

Most parents and health professionals found it acceptable, and it reassured many mothers at home with low scoring babies that urgent medical attention was not required. It also enabled them to identify serious illness and take appropriate action. This is an elegant example of a scientific study designed to identify the best predictors of serious illness and to enable mothers to use this information to decide how seriously ill their babies are.

Cardiovascular risk

How effective is screening for cardiovascular risk factors and appropriate interventions in general practice? Results of two large evaluations of health checks and interventions for cardiovascular risk factors from general practice suggest that the impact on public health is likely to be marginal.[45]

Primary care alone is not going to produce large reductions in the risk of cardiovascular disease. The Government needs to support more effective health policies on tobacco control and healthy eating. Given the proven success of simple interventions in reducing mortality in those already diagnosed as having cardiovascular disease, and the high prevalence of proved cardiovascular disease in the population, practice nurses may be more effectively used with patients at established high risk.[6]

There seems little justification for the ritualistic collection of risk factors when the public health benefits are marginal. The voluntary health promotion package in primary care cannot be justified in its present form, and alternative preventive strategies need to be developed and evaluated. The ethics of screening seem to have been ignored in the new contract imposed on GPs.[7]

Conclusion

Risk is inherent in most treatments and all behaviours. How much is acceptable will depend on the nature of the problem, the acceptability of alternative options and outcomes, and the willingness of doctors to share information about risk with patients, managers, and politicians.

1 BMA Report. *Surrogacy: ethical considerations*, London, BMA, 1990.
2 Morley C, Thornton A, Cole T, Hewson P. Interpreting the symptoms and signs of illness in infants. *Recent advances in paediatrics*, Edinburgh, Churchill Livingstone, 1990: chap 9.

3 Morley C, Thornton A, Cole T, Hewson P, Fowler M. Baby Check: a scoring system to grade the severity of acute systemic illness in babies under 6 months old. *Arch Dis Child* 1991;**66**:100–6.

4 Imperial Cancer Research Fund OXCHECK Study Group. Effectiveness of health checks conducted by nurses in primary care: results of the OXCHECK study after one year. *BMJ* 1994;**308**:308–12.

5 Family Heart Study Group. Randomised controlled trial evaluating cardiovascular screening and intervention in general practice: principal results of British family heart study. *BMJ* 1994;**308**:313–20.

6 Stott NCH. Screening for cardiovascular disease in general practice. *BMJ* 1994;**308**:285–6.

7 Burke P. The ethics of screening. In *Screening and surveillance in general practice* (Hart CR, Burk P, eds), Edinburgh, Churchill Livingstone, 1992:35–44.

34 Urgency

In general practice, accurate assessment of urgency is more important than an accurate diagnosis. Perceptions of urgency affect many decisions made by patients and health professionals. It has social, psychological, cultural, and medical dimensions, and its assessment is a much neglected area of teaching.

Case 200

On 24 December a woman aged 50 presents with a hard painless lump in the breast. She has no past history of breast lumps or serious illness. She is very worried about this. What is your management?

This is the worst time of the year as normal services do not exist within the National Health Service from about 18 December until 2 January. What factors should be considered when urgency is assessed in this case. The mental stress is very great and a diagnosis should be made as soon as possible (125).

> Investigations for patients with suspected malignancy are urgent and should be organised as quickly as possible　　[125]

Should the GP attempt to aspirate this lump? (143)

> Aspiration of a breast lump can be diagnostic and undertaken in the surgery　　[143]

If the GP is not able to do this, the surgical registrar could be asked to see her in the accident and emergency department. This lump was aspirated in the surgery. She was very relieved when clear fluid was removed and the lump disappeared.

Case 201

On 23 December a man aged 59 comes to see you. He was fit until a week ago when he suddenly developed severe pain radiating down the left leg after pushing his car. He said it felt like something tearing. Although the severe pain only lasted for 30 minutes he has developed "cramp" on walking more than 30 yards in the left leg which is relieved by rest. This has never happened before. On examination, the femoral pulse was diminished on the left but the feet were warm and of normal colour. What is your management?

| Accurate assessment of urgency is a prerequisite to effective management [24] |

Did he sprain a muscle and then develop recent intermittent claudication? Assessment of urgency will affect how further investigations are organised (24).

| Urgency is assessed by considering the natural history of the condition, the probability of future complications, the severity of present disabilities, and physical, mental, social, and occupational factors [53] |

In assessing urgency many factors need to be considered (53).

The sudden onset of severe intermittent claudication could be the result of partial arterial occlusion. This could be critical if the blockage becomes complete. This is the worst time of year to get urgent investigations done. What should be done if he intends to go away for Christmas? (431)

| Sudden onset of intermittent claudication needs urgent investigation [431] |

The vascular registrar was telephoned and agreed to see the patient in the outpatient clinic that afternoon. Three weeks later the patient came to the surgery to say how much better he was after his operation. He said that the surgeon was astonished that he had come to the hospital by bus. He had a large dissecting aortic aneurysm which was operated on the same afternoon. Failure to examine this patient's abdomen nearly cost him his life. Fortunately he was saved by good judgement on the assessment of urgency.

Case 202

A woman aged 47 presents with a four month history of stress incontinence. Urine leaks away if she strains, runs, or laughs. It has got much worse over the last two months. On examination she has a prolapse. What is your management?

| The severity of a problem and its disability should be assessed in functional, psychological, occupational, social, and sexual terms [176] |

What factors need to be considered in assessing the severity of this problem? (176)

A knowledge of hospital waiting lists affects the way urgent investigations, appointments, and referrals are organised, and should precede selection of place of referral [126]

Before deciding where to refer a patient for surgery, information is needed about: • waiting times for clinic appointment • waiting times for surgery [564]

The doctor and the patient may not share the same perception of what is urgent or is an emergency [236]

When making an outpatient referral, the GP must indicate the urgency and severity of the problem [317]

This is a most distressing, embarrassing, and disabling complaint. The patient should be referred to a gynaecologist with a special expertise in this condition. Waiting lists will, however, also affect the decisions about place and method of referral (216). Information is needed about two sorts of waiting lists (564).

There may be a three month wait for an outpatient clinic appointment followed by a one month wait for surgery. Alternatively the patient may get an appointment within two weeks, followed by a wait of 18 months for surgery.

When these factors have all been considered, how does the doctor's assessment compare with that of the patient? (236)

Social embarrassment is severe and justifies the request for urgent assessment and treatment. This must be clearly stated in the referral letter (317). Most consultants read the referral letters and will decide on urgency on the basis of information provided by the GP.

Case 203

A man aged 32 who is a known asthmatic comes to surgery 5.25 p.m. with an exacerbation of wheezing and cough. He sees your partner and is given antibiotics and a course of prednisolone. At 6.20 p.m. his wife telephones to ask for a doctor to visit as his breathing is worse. The call is put through to you as you are the duty doctor. You ask if he could be brought back down to the surgery in a car and she says that she will try. Fifteen minutes later the receptionist tells you that they have telephoned to say a 999 ambulance is coming so a visit will not be necessary. What is your response?

The GP has a responsibility to do an immediate visit on any patient after a 999 call has been made, and to provide emergency treatment if needed while waiting for the ambulance [342]

This man was seen in surgery one and a half hours ago. A 999 ambulance has been sent for and the visit was cancelled. Does anything further need to be done? His condition has obviously deteriorated since being seen in surgery. The patient's condition may now be critical (342).

If the ambulance is delayed he could die without any emergency treatment being given. An immediate visit was done. The patient was pale, sweating, and dyspnoeic. The chest was silent. He was critically ill. The ambulance took another 20 minutes to arrive. In the meantime emergency treatment was given and a letter written. The hospital registrar was telephoned to inform her of his condition and imminent arrival.

Case 204

You visit a man aged 68 who has been discharged home following an angiogram done to investigate intermittent claudication. His foot has become cold and painful since the angiography two days ago, but the colour is normal. You discuss this with surgical registrar. A partial arterial embolism or thrombosis is suspected. He says that there are no beds today but he will try to get him in tomorrow for streptokinase treatment. What is your management?

Assessment of urgency based on first hand observation of patient is of more value than assessment by people who have not seen the patient [403]

Good management in general practice depends upon accurate judgement of severity and urgency. Discussions with hospital colleagues often help to identify appropriate management, but the initial assessment of urgency is the responsibility of the GP (403).

When perceptions of urgency differ between GP and hospital specialist, it is the GP's assessment that should affect management decisions outside hospital [404]

The GP is also responsible for ensuring that optimal treatment is obtained for the patient. Is there a difference in perceptions of urgency here? (404)

Once optimal management has been identified, bed availability in one hospital must not be the determinant of management strategy [405]

The decision to admit a patient to hospital is affected by differential diagnosis, probability of serious disease or complications, assessment of disability and urgency, need for hospital tests and treatment, resources at home and in the community, social and family circumstances, psychological factors, doctor's skills, willingness to undertake home care, use of deputising service, and acceptability to patient and family [96]

When demand for a test (or treatment) exceeds available resources, for example, investigation of angina, criteria for assessing risk are needed, based on factors such as age, smoking, BP, occupation, dependants, lipids, family history and past history, presence of chronic disease, severity of disability, and other observations that correlate with a positive test [512]

In this case, an accurate assessment of urgency may be critical. The rest pain is the result of partial arterial occlusion and any delay could result in amputation (405, 96).

To save this limb, every effort must be made to get this patient admitted immediately for streptokinase treatment.

Case 205

A woman aged 49, obese and a non-smoker with five children, develops anginal type chest pain for one week. On examination there are no abnormal findings. Chest radiograph and electrocardiogram are normal. You feel that she needs an urgent exercise electrocardiogram to establish diagnosis. The cardiology senior registrar says that they are overloaded with requests for this test. He suggests treatment with a β-blocker, aspirin, and isosorbide. If this relieves the pain he suggests referral to the cardiology clinic. What thoughts do you have about dealing with the overwhelming demand for this investigation?

There are four aspects to this problem. The first relates to perceptions of urgency. The goal is to prevent a coronary and if she has angina she may need urgent angioplasty or surgery. The second concerns the criteria used to ration such investigations among patients with the same clinical needs. The third factor is the number of coronary bypass operations purchasers have agreed to fund. Finally there is an ethical issue about what happens to patients who need surgery when there are no more funds available until the new financial year?

The registrar's dilemma highlights the need to develop rationing criteria for investigations which may lead to lifesaving treatment. The health service has always been best used by higher socioeconomic groups. First come first served is not an equitable way to allocate scarce resources (512).

The factors in rule 512 need to be weighed alone and in combination, and adjusted for the total amount of resources available to deal with patients whose test is positive. Very few hospitals wish to develop explicit rationing criteria.

Criteria for undertaking an investigation should be:

- jointly drawn up by hospital staff and GPs
- based on best available evidence
- tested to ensure that it only generates enough patients for whom there are facilities
- make available to all GPs
- revised when resources and priorities change or new information is available

[513]

Recent onset of angina needs urgent referral for investigations to determine whether angioplasty or surgery is indicated to prevent a coronary thrombosis [466]

Each of these issues needs to be tackled individually. Drawing up criteria for the allocation of priorities seems to be appropriate. Who, however, should participate in this sort of discussion? Consumers of health services need to be involved in such decisions (513).

Most health service management is a response to crisis because the basic service is underfunded. Politicians have centralised authority and decentralised blame. Managers are reluctant to involve patients in decisions about priorities, and doctors have to make critical choices between different patients whose clinical needs are similar.

The great advantage of making criteria explicit is that all can see what medical, social, epidemiological, psychological, and functional criteria are used for making rationing decisions. Such a process can help to make decisions about who should receive urgent treatment. The purchasers may, however, have underestimated the number of patients who need such investigations and treatment. This issue needs to be discussed jointly by purchasers and providers.

This patient needs urgent investigations. The subsequent availability of surgery is a separate issue. One option is to request an extra contractual referral which would certainly be appropriate in this case (466).

She is young and has five children. After discussion with the consultant a thallium scan was done in view of her obesity.

Conclusion

Different people have different perceptions of urgency. We must try to resolve the patients', GPs', and hospital colleagues' perceptions in a way that is acceptable to all within the constraints of available resources.

35 Social problems

Social factors form the hub around which management decisions revolve in general practice. They are powerful determinants of morbidity and mortality. They also affect the acceptability of treatment and the ability of families to care for relatives. Social interactions, work difficulties, redundancy, unemployment, and housing problems form the context within which illness presents itself in general practice.

Case 206

A man aged 62 is seen in surgery for acute bronchitis. He wonders if you ought to visit his daughter. No one apart from the parents has seen her for 30 years. She is very disabled and is unable to walk or talk or do anything for herself. You visit and find her clean, paralysed, incontinent with fixed flexed limbs, and cared for in a cot. They have an old metal wheelchair which she sits in during the day. The parents seem to be managing well and do not want to leave her or have her put in a home or a hospital. They do not want respite care. What do you do?

> The disability of an illness is assessed by its effects on relatives as well as on the patient [68]

> The management of disability, chronic disease, and malignancy is based on assessment of needs, family's role, and eligibility for financial allowances [70]

> Plans for long term care should be considered when children with learning difficulties or severe physical disabilities are looked after by elderly patients [69]

The parents have provided a lifetime of continuous love and care for their daughter but they are now elderly (68).

Present management includes a full assessment of the physical, social, and psychological needs of patient and parents (70).

The social worker helped them to obtain the disability allowance which can be claimed for retrospectively. The occupational therapist assessed the most suitable aids needed for home care and ensured that these were obtained. One of the long term objectives is to plan ahead (69).

A crisis can be prevented if plans for predictable future events are made now. Long term plans were made with the consultant for patients with learning difficulties. These were activated when the father died a few months later.

Case 207

A woman aged 92 lives alone beyond safe independent existence but is supported by her daughter-in-law. The grandson requests help to save his mother from a mental breakdown as she is no longer able to look after the old woman. You visit and see the patient together with the daughter-in-law. The old woman refuses all offers of help, holidays, or sheltered accommodation, and says that she will be fine while the family are away on holiday. It is obvious that she will not be able to manage. What is your management?

This is a real social emergency and in such cases many alternative options need to be explored (162).

The carer can no longer cope and this has precipitated a social emergency (710). Help might be obtained from respite care but this is only a temporary measure (548).

What place is there for a domiciliary visit by the geriatrician or one of his team? (161)

> In a social emergency, suitable management options may be identified by social worker, health visitor, consultant (domiciliary visit), carers, relatives, neighbours, or voluntary agencies, for example, Cross Roads schemes [162]

> A social emergency occurs when illness in a carer necessitates admission, and urgent help may be needed from community care services, voluntary organisations, for example, Cross Roads, the family, or neighbours [710]

> Respite care is a useful management option for preventing or dealing with social emergencies or family crises [548]

> A domiciliary visit may make certain management options more acceptable to patients [161]

> If a patient needs admission because carer is temporarily unable to cope, consider:
>
> - extra resources at home, for example, day or night sitters, community physiotherapist, Cross Roads schemes, hoists, etc
> - extra resources in the community, for example, day hospitals, day centres, etc
> - respite care rather than admission to acute medical surgical ward   [521]

Acceptability may be influenced by discussion with a hospital specialist or a member of the team for care of elderly people (521).

In this case, a combination of Cross Roads support and help from district nurses, neighbours, and the team for elderly people managed to maintain her home care, while the family had their holiday.

Case 208

A woman aged 82, blind, partially deaf, living in old people's home where there is a warden but no nursing facilities, is looked after by her family who call every day and try to help. They put her to bed each night at 8.30 p.m. She has a commode and often falls when trying to use it. Six weeks ago she had a coronary from which she made a good recovery. She now has the beginnings of a bed sore. Her son telephones to say that the warden telephoned him saying that his mother should really be in hospital as she needs care at night and cannot cope alone. What is your response?

> Elderly people with a medical, psychiatric, or social emergency or problem should not be admitted to hospital before evaluation of the effects of maximum community care services   [182]

The son is giving you the warden's assessment. This may be accurate but should it form the basis for your own management decision? A professional assessment of need should precede decisions about long term care (182).

Is this patient receiving all the community support services that she needs? Is she getting the disability allowance that would enable her to buy in more help? (96)

> The decision to admit a patient to hospital is affected by differential diagnosis, probability of serious disease or complications, assessment of disability and urgency, need for hospital tests and treatment, resources at home and in the community, social and family circumstances, psychological factors, doctor's skills, willingness to undertake home care, use of deputising service, and acceptability to patient and family   [96]

Can the GP assess this patient's needs or would a joint assessment with the district nurse or the occupational therapist be more useful? The community care services could be asked to assess and discuss their findings with you afterwards. Do voluntary organisations have a place in the management of this kind of patient?

Case 209

A woman aged 70 is a likeable late onset dropout, who has neglected herself. She is dirty and smelly. Her toe nails curl over, her feet are filthy, and she dribbles urine. She is not demented or confused. She refuses all forms of help. She is content to remain as she is. The social worker and her neighbours are, however, unhappy. The home help and bath attendant refuse to go in. Meals on wheels leave food outside the front door. Her flat is a shambles. The social worker thinks that there may be a remedial cause for her incontinence but she refuses to be examined. What is your management?

What factors need to be considered here? Is she really a danger to herself? Is she competent to decide to reject help? Being smelly, incontinent, and dirty does not constitute a threat to life. She seems mentally competent and quite content. Doing nothing may be acceptable to the patient and her GP, but not to others involved in providing support and services (539).

Has the point of trying all options been reached or could other colleagues suggest options that the GP may have overlooked? (555)

The decision that nothing more can be done is made at one point in time. People change their minds (49). It must be remembered that she is competent to consent or refuse treatment (50).

She accepted the offer of a weekly bath at the health centre and on one memorable occasion she had a domiciliary consultation with the geriatrician while having a bath. She was also able to have chiropody treatment at the health centre.

> It is important to identify when all available options have been offered and refused, or tried and failed, and where nothing further can be done at the present time [539]

> In a medical, social, or psychiatric emergency, joint consultation with other key personnel and agencies may help to identify suitable management options [555]

> Management decisions are based on needs and acceptability which change over time [49]

> Informed consent is needed for doing nothing, which should be a decision made by the patient after being informed of the possible outcomes, and the effectiveness and acceptability of all other options [50]

Case 210

A social worker tells you that she has just visited a single parent aged 19, because neighbours say that she leaves her child aged three years alone in the house. The mother admits that she does leave the child alone, but only for a couple of hours while she goes out to do her daily shopping. The child seems clean and well nourished. She is a new patient to the practice and you have not seen her. The social worker asks for your opinion on further management. What do you suggest?

> It may be necessary to obtain urgent information about new or temporary patients from previous GP, other hospitals, or social services department [594]

> Patients with chronic illness, long term disability, or social or psychological problems should be informed about voluntary or self help groups [332]

Is a visit indicated? If, so, what could be achieved? Management decisions should be postponed until more information is obtained. This is a new patient (594).

The social worker could find out if this family were known to the social services in the district where she had previously been living. She could also find out whether the child has ever been on the child protection register. Would it be useful to contact her previous doctor? When more information has been obtained, it becomes easier to assess risk and plan appropriate follow up (332).

Single parents need more help and it may be useful to put her in touch with local Gingerbread or Newpin groups.

Case 211

A woman aged 22 comes to surgery and is very depressed. Three months ago she had a stillbirth at 33 weeks. She is a single parent and, although she does not have a stable relationship and lives alone, she wanted the baby very much. There were no avoidable factors in this stillbirth and postmortem examination showed no abnormalities. She is very angry with the hospital because she says that they agreed to pay for the funeral but when she received the bill from the undertakers the hospital said that she had to pay it herself. The hospital midwives were contacted and said that she had been given a choice between a burial by the hospital or one paid for by herself in which she would have a headstone. She does not remember being given any choice and now has a funeral bill of £250 which she is unable to pay. She does have a job but now has total debts of £600. She is very depressed about her financial problems. What is your management?

Financial problems incurred by hospital management decisions may be clarified by discussions with the relevant business manager [680]

Financial problems related to illness may sometimes be alleviated by discussions with voluntary organisations and relevant charities [681]

People with financial problems need information about debt lines and financial counselling services which exist in many districts [682]

Can the GP identify ways in which the finanical debts can be reduced? (680) Some options are not always considered by GPs (681).

She has other financial problems for which help and advice are needed (682).

After discussing the misunderstanding with the relevant hospital manager, it was agreed that the hospital would meet the funeral bill.

Conclusion

Social factors are not always apparent but should always be considered when patients present with symptoms suggestive of stress, anxiety, or depression.

Acceptability, compliance, perceptions of illness, disability, and home care should always be examined within the relevant social context. When this is done, management will be more appropriate, feasible, acceptable, and effective.

36 Conclusion

Just as machines have built in obsolescence, so decisions have built in fallibility. A very wide range of knowledge is needed to make safe and effective decisions. Our roles and responsibilities are changing all the time and we must learn to work in an environment in which constant change is the only certainty. This means that decision making skills become more important than ever.

General practice is one of the most intellectually demanding specialties in medicine. The problems analysed in this book show the enormous range of decisions that need to be made by the GP. Doctors often need to make decisions quickly. It is not necessary to reinvent the wheel each time. Clinical experience helps us to make more effective decisions, and students and young doctors can capitalise on the experience of others. I hope that the study of these cases and the relevant rules might be one way of doing this.

The methods of decision support presented in this book are in their infancy. This approach can be refined and its applications extended, and is an exciting and rewarding field of study. The software program being developed should help students and doctors to explore the rule base for help in making decisions about the management of a wide range of problems seen in daily practice.

At the end of the consultation your judgement will determine what is or is not done. Decision making skills can ensure that this judgement is sound and appropriate for the circumstances at the time. This is a reasonable expectation and one that should help to ensure safe and acceptable patient care in general practice.